GREETINGS My African American Sisters and Women of All Colors:

Are you taking care of yourself? Are you keeping up on your health? Are you having your annual physicals like you should?

In particular, are you taking care of your breasts? Yes, I said breasts. They need very special attention you know. Why? Because a lump can start to form there and grow for years without you knowing it, until one day you feel it. That's why it's very important to have timely mammograms according to your age. Having a mammogram can result in detecting lumps at a very early stage, even before you or your doctor can feel them. Having mammograms when you should, could save your life one day.

It's also important to conduct self-breast exams to determine if there are any changes in your breasts that would require contacting your doctor **_before_** your annual physical is due.

According to the American Cancer Society, breast cancer is the second major cause of cancer death in women. The most recent data shows that mortality rates are falling in Caucasian women, but not in African American women. It is believed that the

T5-DHA-400

(over)

decline in whites may be due to earlier detection and improved treatment. The higher death rate among African American women is believed to be due to finding breast cancer at a late stage.

Go ahead, don't be hesitant. Please take time out for yourself. Keep your mind at ease. Make sure your body gets the special treatment it deserves - keep it **HEALTHY,** for you and your family!

And sisters, if you love your fellow sisters, when in conversation, remember to ask them if they have had their annual mammogram. Believe me when I tell you; ***this is an act of love***.

Why am I saying all of these things? Because we all need to be reminded from time to time of what's **REALLY** important - our health!

AND. . .because if the story I'm about to tell can influence YOU in deciding to have a mammogram when needed, and practice self-breast exams, I will consider it all worthwhile. . . READ ON!

FINDING COMFORT IN THE "Z O N E"

**Encouragement for Healing and Deliverance
for
Women Diagnosed with Breast Cancer**

According to Webster's dictionary, a ZONE is a distinctive area set apart for a particular purpose. Whatever "zone" you find yourself in, try to determine what God wants you to do while you're in it, and most importantly, remember that God can see you through it.

My story was written and produced by the Holy Spirit. I pray God approves of the purpose of this book. I have poured my heart and soul into it. I don't think I have ever had such focus laid upon my spirit. Thank you for using my mind, soul, and spirit Lord. Guide my hands as your tool. Please continue to use me. I'm not tired yet.

**by
Sheila A. Stover, RT. RM.
An African-American
Mammographer/Writer**

First Edition
1 2 3 4 5 6 7 8 9 10

Published by:
S.A.S., Inc.
2883 Farmington Circle, SW
Canton, OH   44706
(330) 478-1632

Library of Congress Catalog Card Number:
ISBN 0-9659846-0-5

Printed in the United States of America

S.A.S., Inc.

To order copies of this book, please write or contact the publisher below:

Published by:
S.A.S., Inc.
2883 Farmington Circle, SW
Canton, OH   44706
(330) 478-1632

LORD, I WANT TO HIDE

Lord, the book is finished.
I just want to hide behind your light of glory.
Lord, just let me hide.
Let your blessings glisten.
Behind your shining light, move in a mighty way Jesus.
Hide me behind your light.
Jesus is the Author and Finisher of the book,
"Finding Comfort in the Zone."
Just take a look as you flip the pages.
Just watch God shine.
Lord, I just want to hide!!
Thank you for sharing and saving my life!

SAS

January 31, 1997

"He must increase, but I must decrease." (John 3:30)

DEDICATIONS

This book is dedicated to all the women who encouraged me through my illness. To my family and friends who did all they could to help. To my husband and children, who were a constant reminder that I definitely had something to live for. But most of all, to my Lord and Savior Jesus Christ, who saw fit to sustain me.

THANK YOU JESUS!

P.S. To Mrs. Minnie Hopkins who allowed me to see her strength while battling breast cancer. I love your play area for disabled children. God bless you! (Minnie Hopkins is a principal at Lathrop Elementary School in Canton, Ohio.

Recipe for Completing
'Finding Comfort in the Zone'

Listening to God's call

Open sharing from Sheila

Valuable editing from Cynthia

Each heart that gladly gave

COMMENTS ABOUT
'FINDING COMFORT IN THE ZONE'

Consider it all joy. . . when you encounter various trials.
Knowing that the testing of your faith produces endurance.
And let endurance have its perfect result, that you may be
perfect and complete, lacking in nothing (James 1:2-4)

With Sheila's contribution, our thoughts can and will be more
positive to deal with the day-to-day struggles and pains of life.
Sheila's words and selected prayers touched my heart and soul
when I needed it most. I believe it will do the same for many
others.

Sheila, thank you for caring and sharing this with me.

Dr. Kenneth Nazinitsky
Radiologist

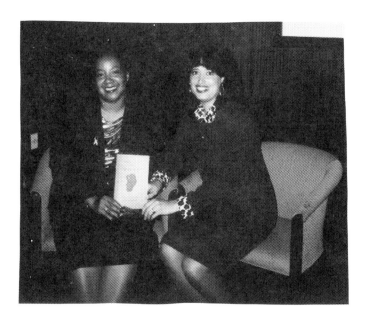

Be encouraged, believe in Jesus Christ.

Rest in God's Word.

Everlasting Life.

Assurance that God is always present.

Scars are a sign of strength.

Treasure every moment of life.

Challenge your body to get well.

Always trust the Lord.

Never give in to Satan.

Conquer this disease.

Each day is a gift from God.

Recovery is possible.

Sheila Stover, RT. RM.
Breast Cancer Survivor
August, 1996

Thought For Every Day

"Don't <u>WASTE</u> your time worrying."

Jesus shed too much blood at the Cross. Allow Him to take
on your fears. He already knew you would be afraid.

<u>Reasons for not fearing:</u>

You are HIS creation!

("Thus saith the Lord that MADE thee,
and FORMED thee from the womb,
which will HELP thee. . ."
Isaiah 44:2)

He FIGHTS for YOU so you can remain AT PEACE!

("The LORD shall fight for you,
and ye shall hold your peace."
Exodus 14:14)

You are LOVED!

("In this was manifested the love of God toward us,
because that God sent his only begotten Son into the world,
that we might live through him."
I John 4:9)

S.A.S.

"FINDING A LUMP"

Christmas, 1993 was a good day. I had been preparing for weeks getting ready for the holidays and enjoying the hustle and bustle of the season. My three children were steadily telling me what they would like to have and I was continually working and shopping to try and make sure their expectations were met. I had to work the afternoon shift on Christmas, so our family dinner was not the usual Christmas dinner. I went to work and things were busy as usual, but it helped the night go fast. Now that Christmas had come and gone, I was already looking forward to what I thought would be a happy New Year.

New Year's Day started out with my husband and I waking to three children who decided they needed to relax and watch early morning TV with us in our bed. After awhile, I had enough and started sending everyone off for their baths.

As I was lying in bed, the phone rang. Aaron, my youngest son, had placed the phone on the floor on my husband's side of the bed. This did not make me happy at the time. As it turned out, making me reach for the phone was truly one of those blessings in disguise.

I rolled from my side to Tony's and when I reached for the phone, I felt something under my right arm. I said to myself, "Oh my, what is this?" As soon as I touched it, I panicked. It was a lump. My husband was lying beside me. He watched me continually palpating this lump, but he didn't ask any questions. I could tell that he was worried because I knew he could feel my panic.

Deep inside of me, I knew what it was immediately because, GUESS WHAT, I'm a Mammography Technologist in the Radiology Department at a local hospital in Canton, Ohio. Yes, I know you're probably wondering why I didn't find this sooner. Of all people, I, a Mammography Technologist, should **<u>KNOW</u>** what to look for!

I had a very sneaky lump - it was deep in my armpit. When I stretched my arm to get the phone, this revealed the lump to me. Thank you Jesus, for my baby boy Aaron!

Children are a gift from the Lord! (Psalms 127:3-5)

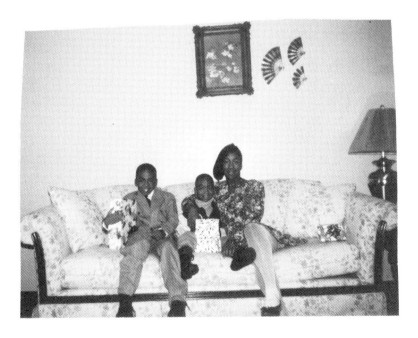

"ACTING UPON MY FINDINGS"

I kept trying to put "the lump" out of my head until I got to work, but it was continually on my mind. On Sunday afternoon, I went to visit my cousin Lydia. She and I sat and talked and enjoyed eating sauerkraut together. I told her I had a lump under my right arm and I needed to get it checked. She encouraged me to make sure I took care of it right away.

Yes, Lydia was right; the most important factor at this point was not to waste time. The easy thing to do would be to deny the fact that I felt the lump. Since the holiday fell on the weekend, I had to wait until Tuesday to get a mammogram. I had a mammogram at age 35 and at this time, I was 38 years old.

I went to work on Tuesday with one thing on my mind: _**"I need help to survive!"**_ When I arrived, Cathy, a fellow Tech on day shift was still there. At the time, I didn't realize what an important role she would play during this crisis in my life.

I asked Cathy to help me take x-rays of the area in question. She immediately was willing to help. I stood at the X-omat (developer) with Cathy, hoping against hope that this thing wouldn't be what I really knew was true. As the films came out, I caught them in my hand - I had breast cancer. I noticed the density (white area) on the films, which left no doubt of full blown breast cancer. At this point, my mind went blank and I think I pretended it was someone else. As with any other patient, we took the films to the darkroom. As I routinely do, I began marking the films with a yellow marking pencil that I use to denote questionable areas for our radiologist to view -- there was no question.

Cathy said, "Oh Sheila, no this can't be happening." We then took the films and went to find a radiologist, who immediately ordered an ultrasound to see if the mass was solid. It was and it measured approximately two centimeters.

The worst part of my night was about to begin - I had to perform my duties as a technologist. After just finding out that I would probably have surgery soon, there were ten women waiting for me to perform their mammograms. But Jesus was with me. I made it through the evening with God's grace. I was able to perform my tasks without shedding a tear.

"Peace I leave with you, my peace I give unto you: not as the world giveth, give I unto you. Let not your heart be troubled, neither let it be afraid." John 14:27

As my night was winding down, I saw Dr. R., our Head Radiologist crossing the main hallway of the X-ray Department. He's one of those people who's always in a hurry; however, when I called him, he came right away. He later told me that he could tell in my voice that I needed his assistance. I showed him my films and he said, "Are these your films?" I responded yes. He said, "You know you need to see a surgeon." Then he said, "I'll be right back." Dr. R. soon returned with an appointment for me the next morning. He had gone to his office and called one of our best local surgeons. As he turned and walked away, although his professional stature was showing, his feelings of concern were visible to me. Dr. R.'s kindness and concern for me will always be greatly appreciated. I needed his assurance.

". . .I am with you always, *even* unto the end of age." Matthew 28:20

"TELLING YOUR SPOUSE"

By now, I still hadn't found time to cry. I kept wanting to just fall apart, but something within me said, "Don't worry, you have lots more work to do." Before Dr. R. left, he suggested I finish my mammogram as I had just x-rayed the affected side. So, I called on another Tech, Angie, who is dear to me. When I showed her my films, we both cried, but I knew she cared about me and it made it easier to do.

After I settled down, I called Tony to tell him we had a Big Problem. I explained what was going on and told him I had to see a surgeon the next morning. He said, "I was wondering when you were going to tell me." He had noticed me checking this area constantly in our bedroom and he knew something was wrong. I told him I was leaving soon and he said he would wait up for me so we could talk. When I got home, we got into bed and we talked. Tony held me tighter than ever before because we were both afraid for our lives and the lives of our children - Tiana 12, Adrian 8, and Aaron 3. All I could think of was every mother's prayer, "Lord, please let me live to raise my children. Please don't take me now."

"Trust in the Lord with all thine heart; and lean not unto thine own understanding. In all thy ways acknowledge him, and he shall direct thy paths." (Proverbs 3:5-6)

"MEETING THE SURGEON"

Morning came and we had a blizzard. I called the doctor's office to confirm my appointment. The receptionist said, "Are you coming out in this weather?" I replied, "Yes, I have to keep this appointment."

The roads were terrible, but we made it. I met with Dr. Y. He knew this was definitely something to be concerned about, yet he kept trying to encourage me. He said, "Sheila, we are going to take care of this." We will do a biopsy on January 10th." But I knew all along what needed to be done. Things were moving right along, thank God, but I was absolutely scared at this time.

"For God hath not given us the spirit of fear; but of power, and of love, and of a sound mind." (II Timothy, 1:7)

"RESULTS FROM THE BIOPSY"

January 10th   ---   Biopsy

January 11th   ---   What I thought was doom's day.

On January 11th, I returned to Dr. Y.'s office to get the results of my biopsy. As he checked my incision, he sat me up. At that time, I asked the Big Question - "What was it?" He sat on the stool and started talking. All I heard was, "Something, something, carcinoma." My mind went blank. I felt like I couldn't breathe. I couldn't hear another word Dr. Y. was saying. I could see his lips moving, but I couldn't hear a word. I put my hand up and asked for my husband. He went to get Tony.

Now was my moment of turning into the hysterical patient. By the time Tony entered the room, the reality of this whole crisis had sunk in and I was crying hysterically. I kept repeating to my husband, "I'm sorry, I'm sorry, I'm sick, very sick." He tried to comfort me while holding back his tears.

As they tried to calm me down, I could hear Dr. Y. in the background saying, "Sheila, we can help you, this isn't the end. In the midst of my hysterical fit, Dr. Y. started to talk about having surgery and he gave me two choices: a lumpectomy, which I basically had with the biopsy. It entailed going back to surgery for more node removal - removing lymph nodes under my right arm to check for possible spread of the cancer, and then determining treatment. Or, I could have the "ever-loving mastectomy." He said, "We'll wait two weeks and then you can decide."

All of a sudden, I came to myself and said, "No, I can't wait two weeks. You call someone and tell them I'm coming next week and I want a mastectomy - just take it off. I don't want it." Dr. Y. agreed. Tony said, "Sheila, are you sure?" I replied, "Yes, my kids are too young. I want it off. Just throw it away." Thank God for a strong will!

"I WILL lift up mine eyes unto the hills, from whence cometh my help." (Psalms 121:1)

PS: **Please remember that the decision to have a mastectomy was my personal choice. There are other options. If you are faced with this decision, please take time to discuss all your options with your doctor.**

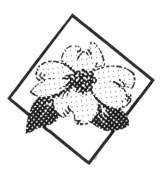

"EMOTIONS"

During the next week, I went through every emotional mood swing. I couldn't go back to work because I just couldn't deal with performing mammograms.

First on the agenda was telling my parents of whom I am the only child they have living. I had a brother who died of a sickness at the age of 25. All I could think of was that God surely wouldn't take me from my family now. My parents had already had such an emotional loss when my brother Adrian passed away in 1972.

When I told them, my heart started beating wildly. The lump in my throat was so big, I felt as though I could hardly swallow or talk. I just couldn't tell them how bad I knew this could be, but I didn't have to - they knew themselves. I needed both of them to be strongholds for me and my family. This was very hard for them. The first thing my mother said was, "I wish I could do this for you." I could see the pain on my dad's face. Thank you Lord, for my parents, a constant stronghold.

"In every thing give thanks: for this is the will of God in Christ Jesus concerning you." (I Thessalonians 5:18)

NOTE: Make sure that you understand what this scripture **REALLY** means. It is God's will that you give Him thanks **IN EVERYTHING** or **THROUGH EVERYTHING**. In other words, are you able to say that in spite of your circumstances, you can still give God thanks?

"GETTING READY FOR SURGERY"

I went to surgery on Wednesday, January 19, 1994. It was the coldest day ever - 26 degrees below zero. We got in the car at 5:00 a.m. It didn't want to go and neither did I.

My Aunt Betty had spent the night to take care of my children. I love her so much! As I was getting ready to leave, she said something very special to me. She gave me a hug and said, "No tears this morning; you go do what you have to do and everything will be okay. I love you." At that point, Aunt Betty was speaking a gospel to me and I was determined to believe she was right. She's a very special member of my family - my daddy's sister, whom I've always loved dearly. There was no need to worry about my children either - Aunt Betty was there.

**"Therefore I say to you; do not worry about your life."
(Matthew 6:25) His eye is on the sparrow, I know he
watches me. (SAS)**

"THE MAN I MARRIED"

At the time of surgery, I had been married to my husband for 16 years. We had experienced ups and downs like any other marriage. But when this storm got in our way, I met a person that I could love forever. Tony showed a side of himself I had never met. Like most men, he tried hard not to show his emotions. But as we were getting ready to leave for the hospital, we had one of the most tender moments since the birth of our children. He turned out the lights in our bedroom and beckoned me to come to him. He wrapped me in his arms, and held me tight. At that moment, he said, "Let's pray." We both fell to our knees and my husband prayed out loud, beseeching the Lord on my behalf. For me, this was a very touching moment in our lives and I thank God for that moment. Tony's prayer is something I will never forget.

"And God said, Let us make man in our image, after our likeness. . .;" "So God created man in his own image, in the image of God created he him; male and female created he them." (Genesis 1:26, 27)

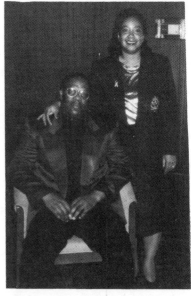

"SURGERY"

As I was separated from my family, I realized; "Jesus, it's me and you. I'm trusting you to guide the surgeon's hands, the nurse's hands, and especially the anesthesiologist's hands. Please don't let me wake up in the middle of surgery (smile)." Aunt Betty's words of no crying came back to me, but I just couldn't help it. Now was the time to cry. Dr. Y. entered the surgery suite, grabbed my hand and winked his eye. All I can remember saying was, "The Lord is my shepherd," and I was fast asleep. Thank God for anesthetic.

The First Anesthetic

"And the Lord God caused a deep sleep to fall upon Adam, and he slept: and he took one of his ribs, and closed up the flesh instead thereof;" (Genesis 2:21)

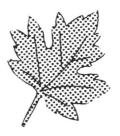

"AWAKING"

When I awoke several hours later, I could hear my husband's voice, but I couldn't see him. Once I was awake, reality set in. My right breast was gone. At this point, my family and friends rallied around me with nothing but love. The hospital personnel were absolutely wonderful. I had received flowers, cards and gifts from many people wanting to show their support and love.

But all of a sudden, I could feel myself sinking into a mood of depression and fear. What's next? Am I going to have to endure chemotherapy? Am I going to lose my hair? Am I going to see my children grow up?

"Lord, please be a fence around me every day."

"LIPSTICK"

Two days after my surgery, I found out that I had four positive lymph nodes, which meant I had to endure chemotherapy. "Panic time" was here. When the Oncologist left, I just buried my head in my husband's chest and cried. I was scared to death.

Two of my most treasured friends, Connie and Bev were waiting outside the door and they could see my pain. When they entered the room, I immediately picked up my lipstick and applied it about four times (I always do this when I'm nervous). Connie can always make me laugh. She said, "Sheila, how many times are you going to put on that lipstick?" In the midst of tears, we found a reason to laugh.

"God sits in heaven and laughs." (Psalms 2:4). "A woman of strength is one who rejoices." (Proverb 31:25)

"MY WORKING MAN"

During my stay in the hospital, before he went to work, my husband would show up at 6:00 a.m. to check on me. I would get up early and try to make myself look nice before he arrived so he wouldn't worry all day at work. As long as I had my lipstick on, he knew I was okay. His love for me was expressed by just showing up so early in the morning. Thank you Lord, for a caring husband.

Miracle of marriage - Two people actually become one flesh (Ephesians 5:23-27).

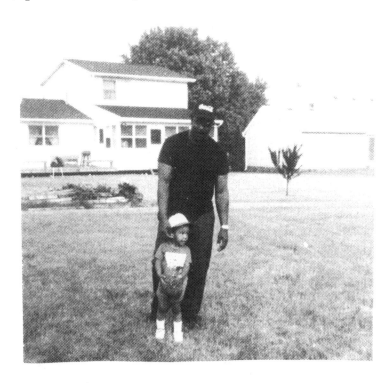

"GOING HOME"

Going home was very scary because I was thinking about all the things that come after surgery.

I nervously went home on Sunday and my recuperation started. Although I was sick, I had a three-year-old who loved me very much and who was also very demanding. He couldn't go to pre-school because we both needed a sitter (smile).

My family, friends, and co-workers, whom I could not have done without, banned together to take care of us. They did a wonderful job. I had a different baby sitter for Aaron and me every day. As I rested, there was always someone there to watch Aaron.

I also had a visiting nurse, who would come several days a week to check on me. Louise became a good friend. I could tell Louise what was hurting me; things I didn't want to tell my family because I didn't want them to worry.

Sometimes a stranger can be your best friend. (SAS)

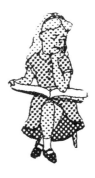

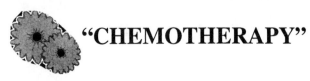 # "CHEMOTHERAPY"

Chemotherapy is a very frightening word. I will never understand this drug, but I thank God for providing something to help extend so many lives, and I'm praying it will sustain my life. When it's mentioned, however, that you need to take this drug, your mind goes 100 miles an hour. It's hard to imagine that you really have a disease that warrants taking a drug you can't understand.

One thing I did learn from taking chemotherapy is that the process of taking this drug is a state of mind. If you concentrate on the fact that it's just an IV, you can handle it much better.

My first chemo treatment was February 21, 1994, the week of Aaron's 4th birthday. I had to be hospitalized for a port a cath placement in my chest. Since I didn't have any veins left to take the chemo, a catheter was placed in my chest to access the chemotherapy.

I was determined all of this would be done and over with so I could get home for Aaron's birthday, February 23rd. Every moment was precious and worth living for because my children and family were so important.

All the fears of chemo were on my mind - sickness, hair loss, and just plain looking sick to everyone. I prayed and asked God to please allow me to look like myself. My biggest fear was looking in the mirror and not looking like myself. He blessed me; I only lost ten pounds.

After this first treatment, though, I went home to a bout of four days of sleeplessness due to nervousness. I was upset because I was afraid and because it was my baby's birthday and I wasn't able to even get out to buy him anything. Tony went out and bought him a wonderful present, but it wasn't like I helped. I was very depressed and by day four, I ended up back at the hospital in the emergency room. After two shots and a good sleep, I promised myself that I would **NEVER** let Satan take over again. I wasn't going to worry. I had to go on. Thank you Jesus for peace of mind.

"Peace Be Still."

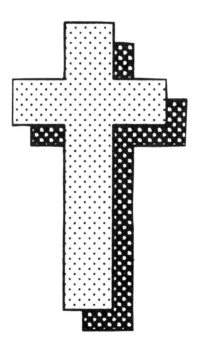

"FAMILY AND FRIENDS"

Family and friends play a big part in the recovery of any patient with a serious illness. If the Lord hadn't blessed me with such a wonderful group of family and friends, recovery would have been much harder - from finances to meals, to baby sitting, to grocery shopping, to doctor visits, to housekeeping, to just talking and keeping my mind off things - I could not have asked for more.

I have a very close friend who is a fellow mammographer. Her name is Dency. She lives several miles from Canton in a town called Waynesburg, Ohio, but she found time in her busy schedule to shop for me and constantly check to make sure I was all right.

I had a major phobia whenever I would go to the hospital for blood work or x-rays. My co-workers meant well, but they would say, "Doesn't she look good!!" This would instantly upset me. I would wonder and think, "Where is their faith? What did they think I was going to look like?"

One day, I explained how I felt to Dency. The next time she saw me at the hospital, she dropped a note in my pocket. It read: I hate your hair, where did you get that awful lipstick. Now that's a friend. She knew my need. Instead of crying that day, I laughed all the way home.

During the course of my illness, two very wonderful pastors stepped in to fill the gap due to the fact that our church was in search of a pastor. A BIG "God Bless You" goes out to Rev. and Mrs. Claybourne Giles and Rev. and Mrs. Cato Waiters. Also, I know that a lot of people don't agree with women being ministers, but Mrs. Edelaide Frazier was a special part of my healing process. The Lord sent her always at the right time. God Bless You Mrs. Frazier. Your quiet ministry was special to me.

**A genuine friend multiplies the joys we share
and divides the sorrows.**

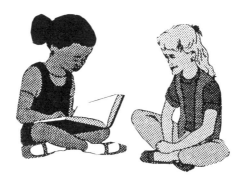

"HAIR LOSS"

"Lord, have mercy Jesus!!!" Ten days after my first chemo treatment, I lost my hair. My sister-in-law, Brenda and I had bought a wig two weeks earlier, so I thought I was ready. No woman is ever ready to lose her hair! It is very important to get a wig before chemo treatment because it will help you feel somewhat prepared.

First, my hair became as hard as an SOS pad. Then it got very brittle about the eighth day after chemo. I went to church, but I was scared to comb it. I was very self conscious about it falling out. On Monday, I woke up and if you touched it, it just fell out. I drove to my friend's house, Rhonda, who is a barber (only your hairdresser knows - smile!). She tried to condition my hair with the best conditioners, but it didn't work. Finally, I said, "Just cut it off." Rhonda was so kind to me. There were no mirrors for me to see her cutting my hair. She then cut the wig I had brought into a wonderful style to fit my face. Rhonda handed me my lipstick and then we went to the mirror. I was upset, but all in all, I looked good (smile). Thank you Jesus, for Rhonda! Afterwards, I knew it was time to move on.

"But the very hairs of your head are all numbered."
(Matthew 10:30) I love the fact that God knows everything about me, even the number of hairs on my head!

"WIG WEARING"

I've always been a woman of variety and when it came to wigs, I ended up with six. One morning my husband woke up, looked over at my dresser where there were six different wigs, all lined up on six wig heads. Tony turned and looked at me and said, "Sheila, I'm not trying to upset you, but how many wigs do you need? Baby, none of them really look like you - but they're all nice." To say the least, I stopped buying wigs.

I lost my hair, but a big, big thank-you goes out to Kim Fields of Living Single (TV show). I was able to get through the wig situation by just watching her character on television. Her variety of changing hair styles with wigs really helped me. I was very self conscious of wearing the wig, but she helped me make a game out of wig wearing. I might have long hair at noon and short hair by 4:00 p.m.

"Variety is the Spice of Life!" Thanks Kim!

"GOING BACK TO WORK"

Since my job consisted of performing mammograms, I had to mentally prepare myself to go back to work. As the kids say, "**In Your Face**," the reality of dealing with breast cancer was definitely in my face - daily.

I spent a lot of time washing my face, fighting back the tears as I x-rayed women day after day. On the evening shift, there's no one to relieve me. I had to stand strong. Thank you Jesus. You allowed me to return to my job conquering the spirit of fear.

". . . Almost thou persuadest me to be a Christian." (Acts 26:28) I must be a witness (like Paul) in the workplace. You don't know like I know what God has done for ME!

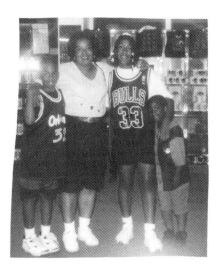

"SCARS"

Scars are a sign of strength. As I look back on how I felt when I first saw my scar, I was deeply hurt. I felt as though I had been robbed of something very precious. It took a long time for me to get past the pain of getting dressed and undressed. We had a large oval mirror in our bathroom. Every time I got out of the shower, no matter which way I turned, I couldn't get away from it. It was always reflecting back that ugly scar.

During this phase in my recovery, I was very bothered by the mirror. Somehow, my mother knew this, and on my birthday that year, my mom and dad bought a new mirror for our bathroom. Tony measured and recessed it into the wall so that when I stepped out of the shower, I could only see from my neck up (smile)!

During this period, I was having many pity parties for myself. On one very special afternoon, God sent me an angel in the form of my 12 year-old daughter, Tiana. I was in one of those moods when I just wanted to hide out in my bedroom where it always felt safe. Tiana and I were lying on the bed and I expressed to her how I felt about the scar. She was quiet for a moment, as though to be deep in thought, and then in a very quiet voice she said, "Mommy, it's only as ugly as you think." That's so true! If I don't think of the scar as ugly - it isn't. Thank you, Lord, for giving my daughter such a wise vision at an early age. Thank you for building my strength through Tiana!

"Out of the mouth of babes often comes wisdom."

"GETTING AWAY"

My advice to any woman who goes through a bout with a serious disease is to get away. I have a lovely friend who is now an ultrasound technologist in Atlanta, Georgia. When I was sick, she flew to Canton to see me.

When Nealy left, she said to me, "Sheila, I want you to come, when you feel better, to visit me in Atlanta. This was a big request, for you see, I 'd never flown before. But I decided to go in August. I took the one hour and seventeen minute flight from Cleveland to Atlanta. Nealy and I had a wonderful time.

One significant thing that happened on this trip was my liberation from my wig. One day, Nealy and I were sitting at the kitchen table. She looked at me and said, "Sheila, I want to see you without your wig. Take it off. Just take that thing off." I immediately grabbed my wig and threw it on the counter. Nealy looked at me and said, "Now that's the Sheila I know." Then Nealy decided to take me shopping. As we worked our way through the crowd, Nealy would point out women with short hairdos. She'd say, "Now look at her; she paid BIG money for that short haircut!"

At Nealy's, I was truly liberated from my wig. After she told me to take it off, I never put it on the remainder of the time I was there. No one knew me or knew what had happened in my life. The freedom I felt there was unbelievable. And all because Nealy told me to "take it off." Thank you Nealy, for the encouragement and the invitation. I love you for caring.

Monday came and it was time to go home. That spirit of fear attacked again. I was very happy without the wig, but I was afraid my family just wasn't ready for the shock. You see, no one but Aaron, my youngest son, had ever seen me without the wig. He was only four at the time. He burst into the bathroom one day and saw me. I told him not to tell and he didn't (smile).

As I was packing, I put the wig back on to come home. When Nealy's husband, Larry, saw me come down the steps, he said, "Sheila, why did you put that wig back on? You looked fine without it." What a support! I explained that my family wasn't ready. In looking back though, I think I was the one who still wasn't yet ready. Larry just smiled and we went to the airport.

However, the freedom I felt in Atlanta, had a bigger impact than I thought. Two days after I got home, I began to tell my family and co-workers to get ready - no more wig wearing for me!

The first couple of days at work, heads were turning, but I was comfortable and at peace with myself. One of the doctors blessed me in the hallway the day after I took the wig off. Dr. R. walked up to me, smiled and said, "Sheila, you have a nice head. If you have to lose your hair, it's good to have a nice head." This was a special complement.

Encouragement is a gift for your hearer.

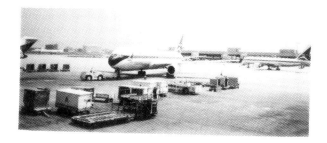

"ADRIAN"

Two and a half years after my surgery, something very special happened. My middle child, Adrian, asked the question, "Mommy, did someone in our family have cancer?" I was stunned by the question, but I knew I needed to give him an answer. I said, "Yes Adrian." He asked, "Who?" I replied, "Me, but God has blessed mommy, I'm all right." He was satisfied with my answer and I was blessed by the fact that he had lived through my storm without a blemish. I feel through this, Adrian has learned to trust God at an early age. I'm very happy he was too young to worry.

Fruit of the Spirit

"Peace" The peace of God protects us from worry and fear. Romans 5:1-11.

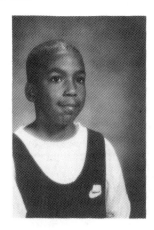

"90 MILE CHECK UPS"

At this point in my recovery, I receive what I call my 90 mile checkups. Protocol for my chemo treatment states that I must see my Oncologist every three months for a checkup.

I am very fortunate to have a wonderful, God-fearing Oncologist. He has the ability to stay cool and calm through many crises.

When I reach the parking lot, I stop and pray before I go in. This is a very nerve racking time for me, but I don't want to miss one visit.

When I turn the corner to go to Dr. M's office, the O from Oncology hits me in the face and I say to myself, "Was I really sick enough to have to come to this department?"

Dr. M. can feel my nervousness when I come in for my 90 mile checkup. When he opens the door to the room I'm waiting in, he immediately starts talking. When he tells me that my blood work looks good, it immediately takes the edge off.

A few 90 mile checkups ago, Dr. M said, "Sheila, this is a maintenance check. You're just stopping by for a quick once over and you're ready to go." Lord, thank You for a praying doctor who's able to feel my need. I'm praying to make it to every maintenance check.

"Yea, though I walk through the valley of the shadow of death, I will fear no evil: for thou art with me; thy rod and thy staff, they comfort me." (Psalms 23:4)

"REACH TO RECOVERY"

Reach to Recovery is an organization through the Cancer Society, which has volunteers who have gone through breast cancer and are willing to share with a woman who recently had surgery.

I received a call in the hospital from a volunteer named Mary. I was very apprehensive to talk with her by myself so I called my husband and asked him to come. He came, and when Mary walked into my hospital room, Tony said, "Hi Mary." She was a friend of his and she was also an African American woman. Although I was a professional worker in the hospital, I was still a very scared woman. During this time, my surgery was only two days old. My arm was in a sling and I was in pain and very scared.

Mary sat down and the first thing she did was raise her affected arm straight up - something I thought I would never do again. Mary's visit was an encouragement to me. Every breast cancer patient needs a "Mary." My Mary came to me saved, sanctified, and filled with the Holy Ghost. Thank You again Jesus!

Faithfulness - Every act done for the Master counts.

"SUPPORT GROUPS"

Support groups can be very beneficial to a woman recovering from breast cancer. In every city, there are groups of women who meet weekly or monthly to encourage each other.

I feel that the main purpose of support groups is to help women realize they are not alone as they talk through their fears.

My support group is through my work. Each day is a challenge as I ask God to help me stand strong in the face of breast cancer daily. I usually don't discuss what happened to me with my patients unless it is someone who has already lost a breast. As I begin to perform the mammogram, I usually say to my patient, "How long ago did you have surgery?" They answer my question and I proceed to tell them I have also lost a breast. At this point, it seems like we both relax because we have something in common. I thank the Lord for the joy and peace He's given me on my job. Many days I'm able to block out my situation and take on the situation of my patient. Thank you Jesus for teaching me to pray for my patients.

Check with your doctor for a local support group.

Recognize God, adore Him, and praise Him. But most of all, THANK HIM! (SAS)

"QUITTING TIME"

At the area hospital where I work, I service mainly the after-work crowd. I start at 4:30 p.m. and work until 9:30 p.m.

Before I go home every night, while cleaning the rooms up for the next day, "It's Prayer Time." I thank God for my life, my family and the skills that He has allowed me to acquire in my work. The mammography unit is an essential tool and can save many of my fellow sisters by detecting breast cancer at an early stage. I'm very careful in prayer to acknowledge God's presence with me daily as I perform my daily tasks.

"Lord, thank you for the knowledge and the patience. Please anoint my efforts." SAS

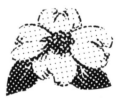

"SPREADING THE WORD"

Every woman, whatever nationality, has a responsibility to encourage her fellow sisters to have regular checkups and annual mammograms. I have a mission of my own now to spread the word in my community where this disease seems to attack daily. In my profession, we deal with cancer and many other diseases daily. Hospital personnel are very special people. We have a very big responsibility to encourage and provide the best care possible.

To my fellow technologists. Take the very best mammograms you can. Sometimes it's hard, but remember, we are the middle person between patient, doctor and diagnosis. The pictures we provide determine each patient's future. This is a huge responsibility. Our patients look to all of us for comfort and assurance, especially when they feel a lump. We are not allowed to give results, but we can always provide an encouraging word.

Trust God for the right words. SAS

"STATISTICS"
(From the Cancer Society)

A mammogram can find breast cancer so small your doctor can't feel.

Research shows that by age 35, a baseline mammogram should be taken. By age 40, mammograms should be taken every two years. After age 50, a mammogram should be taken annually.

If you find a lump, don't waste time. Call your physician right away.

WHEN BREAST CANCER IS FOUND AND TREATED EARLY, THERE IS A 91% SURVIVAL RATE!

Remember, spread the word! Encourage each other!

PS: Remember, I was 38. If you feel the need for a mammogram _anytime_, "GO." Your life could depend on it!

"SELF BREAST EXAM"

Remember to examine your breasts once a month. Ask your doctor, nurse or mammography technologist to teach you the proper method. Be sure to check deep into your armpits and even up into your neck area.

See your doctor for regular breast exams: at least every three years between ages 20 and 40 and every year over 40.

Remember, breast cancer can be very sneaky. Try to stay one step ahead.

Also, if breast cancer hasn't appeared in your family, please don't get caught up into thinking: **"it doesn't run in my family**," therefore, the need to do self breast exams or have mammograms isn't necessary. **Remember, someone must be first.** I was the first in my family to have breast cancer and since my surgery in 1994, two very close family members have also been diagnosed.

Remember to pray. Be encouraged. "SAS"

GOD BLESS!

"PRECIOUS LOVED ONE"
(DeShawn)

My thoughts and prayers are with every one who reads this book. But before I finish, I can't leave out a special thought I had for my loving nephew DeShawn. I would have thought that battling breast cancer was one of the hardest things I would endure. Wrong!! Losing my nephew DeShawn seemed to hurt much much more. May 5, 1995 was one of the worst days. DeShawn, was shot. He lived about six weeks and died on June 11, 1995.

When I awoke from my biopsy, Shawn was the first person I saw. He asked, "Aunt Sheila, are you all right? Are you going to be all right? I replied, "Yes Shawn, I'll be fine."

At that time, I didn't realize Shawn's time was winding up. I miss him dearly and a lot of times, it seems I can feel his presence or hear his voice.

I loved Shawn like one of my children. He wasn't mine by blood, but he was mine in my heart.

When Shawn was taken from us by violence, I couldn't cope with his loss. I refused to go to services. I couldn't bear the reality of what had happened.

About two weeks after the services, I prayed and I told the Lord that I needed to see, hear, and talk to DeShawn. A few nights later, about 4:00 a.m., I woke up, got a drink, and went back to sleep. I began to dream about DeShawn. I saw him lying in the casket. However, at the same time, I could feel him standing behind me. I refused to turn around and look at him. Shawn began to talk to me. He said, "Aunt Sheila, look at me." I replied, "No Shawn, I don't want to look at you."

At my church, we believe God's miracles work in three's and seven's. It took God seven days to finish creation and rest, and three days for Jesus to rise again. Hallelujah! Shawn asked me two more times to turn around and look at him. From this dream, I believe God was telling me, "Though he's dead, you will see him again." While I was looking at him in front of me dead, when I finally turned around, he was standing there very much alive. Shawn said to me, "Aunt Sheila, stop worrying about me. It's fun here!" Thank you God for this dream.

I awoke crying and praising God for this special dream. God gave me just what I asked for. Thank you Jesus. Since this dream, I have comfort in knowing DeShawn's in God's hands.

The poem which brings this book to an end is very special to me. It expresses how I felt. I really can't explain the "zone" I was in when I wrote it, but one thing I do know: we all have to pass through this zone when our lives are over. Shawn has done what we all have to do. Sometimes there is a reason we must leave, but it's on God's time, not our time.

Unconditional love is something Jesus Christ has for all of His children. I thank God for giving me an unconditional love for this very special young man.

Lord when it's time for me to fly, make it a safe flight, straight to Your throne.

Peace and the Love of Jesus Christ Be With You Shawn. Until we meet again.

Aunt Sheila

Mom and Dad, Mr. & Mrs. G., Tony, Tiana, Adrian and Aaron, I Love You - Sheila (Mom) "SAS"

PS: Can't forget Eric and Corey. Love always.

"SHEILA'S PRAYER"

God Almighty, my Lord and Savior, thank You for amazing grace. Thank You for my precious life. With all Your mighty wisdom, You already know my fate. From my mother's womb to my dying hour, I will trust You. My future generations will come and go, You already know each and every one's name and life story.

Guide us Lord, with Your infinite wisdom. Protect my present and future generations from this dreaded disease and anything else which can cause hurt, harm, or danger. I will be ever so careful to give You all the honor and the praise.

AMEN!

PRAYER CHANGES THINGS!

Sheila Stover, RT. RM.
Mammographer
August, 1996

I SHALL NOT DIE,

BUT LIVE,

AND DECLARE

THE WORKS

OF THE LORD!

Psalms 118:17

**Encouragement for Healing and Deliverance
for
Women Diagnosed with Breast Cancer**

GOD ANSWERS
DIFFICULT QUESTIONS

1. Where was God when illness invaded my life? God is
   omnipresent. He knows everything; from past, to your
   present, to your future. Trust Him and you'll feel His
   presence. God *allows* trials to happen, expecting praise
   during and after He delivers our circumstance. (Is. 4:9,10)

2. Lord, when will I heal? Psalms 18:25

3. Lord, will I recover from cancer? (Matthew 19:26) God
   wants you to be healed. (Psalms 18:25)

Some say you never know a woman's strength until she meets a
trial. Breast cancer will make a woman show her strength.
(When the battle is over and the victory is won!) SAS

Sometimes, we focus so much on outward appearance, such as
clothes, jewelry, makeup, and weight, that we forget what's
really important. The Bible states that of all the things a
woman may wear, her expression is the most important. Her
outlook, showing a calm and quiet spirit, will give her peace (I
Peter 3:4).

Her children called her blessed and her husband praised her as
a wonderful woman (Proverbs 31:28-29). Praise from your
family is so important to any woman because they are the ones
who observe you. The praise of your family should encourage
you through every trial. Remember to ask God to order your
steps.

"PRAYER TIME"

1. Tell God you love Him.
2. Ask God to save you and believe He hears you.
3. Ask God for deliverance from this disease.
4. Believe God is in control of your life.
5. Thank God for all He's done.
6. Believe God loves you.
7. Trust God day and night.
8. Believe God will heal your body.
9. Speak healing and deliverance.

Read These Psalms Daily For Peace

If you're afraid - Psalms 27
If you have doubt - Psalms 73
When you are sick - Psalms 6
When you are lonely - Psalms 12

"QUIET TIME"

1. **The Creation of Woman** - Never think of yourself as an afterthought. God had women in mind from the beginning of creation. God said that man alone was not good. Man needed a woman. Genesis 2:18

2. **Blessings Through Illness** - When God allows us to get well after a serious illness, it's a special gift. Remember to praise Him for your good and bad days (Ps. 103:2-5).

3. **Breasts** - I searched high and low in the Bible looking for a word about breasts. My neighbor, Wanda, came to visit one day and brought me these words of encouragement. "Let your fountain be blessed and rejoice with the wife of your youth (These words involved my husband and I). As a loving deer and a graceful doe, let her breasts satisfy you at all times, and always be caught up in her love (Proverbs 5:18,19)." These words were so special to me because most women worry about a change of feelings from their mate. Thank God I have a man who was very sensitive to our situation. Husbands, love your wives for the breasts that she has (or doesn't have). Amen!

4. **Moving up the Ladder to the Next Level** - After going through surgery, treatment, and recovery - that spirit of doubt will creep in. Constantly believe in healing. Our words mean a lot. Remember, when you move to the next level, there's always another devil.

5. **Self Esteem (Scars)** - Remember to hold your head up! Put on your lipstick! You are the same person you were before surgery. You have just finished running one of the largest obstacle courses of life. That spirit of doubt and feeling less than a woman may step in. Put those feelings to rest. Conquer that fear. Scars are a sign of strength. The scar has extended your life and you made it over. Psalms 139 talks about the wonder of your creation, how God knew you from your mother's womb - trust Him!

6. **The Straight and Narrow Road** - During my illness, we were in search of a new pastor. Our previous pastor, Rev. W.C. Henderson, had reached retirement. Many pastors came and went and I never saw or heard any of them speak because I was recuperating. The temperatures were very cold in Ohio. I received a tape of one of the sermons from our tape ministry. This sermon was given by Rev. A. D. Lewis of Mississippi. I had heard the sermon of the broad and narrow roads many times in my church life, but it never had the impact that his sermon brought forth. Rev. Lewis had a very southern speaking voice, a voice of great clarity. When he began to speak, I could feel the power of God in his voice. He began talking about the broad road and how you can find yourself driving a little less careful and making wider turns because life seems much easier there. Then he began talking about the narrow road and how sometimes when you come to an underpass and your load is too high or too wide - something HAS TO COME OFF to ensure your safety. Tears began to flow because I could relate to something having to come off. Lord, thank you for Your Word through Rev. Lewis. Matt. 8:13-14

7. **Hope - After Breast Cancer** - This I recall to my mind. Therefore I have hope. Through the Lord's mercies, we are not consumed because his compassion fails not. They are new every morning. Great is your faithfulness. The Lord is my portion says my soul. Therefore, I have hope in Him! Thank you Pastor Jordan for bringing forth this word Sept. 8, 1996. God's faithfulness is dependable. (Lamentations 3:21-23). John 10:7-18 - He provides refreshment in the difficult experiences of life.

8. **Protect Me Lord** - I have a desire to be like Daniel, to always pray and give thanks to God Almighty, even when things go wrong. I especially had to take time to praise God for chemotherapy. I will never understand this drug, but I thank God for providing something to help extend so many lives, and I'm praying it will sustain my life. Anyone who has taken chemotherapy can relate to Shadrach, Meshach, and Abednego in the fiery furnace, asking God to help them make it through. Remember the question Nebuchadnezzar asked, "Didn't we put three in the furnace?" The counselors answered, "Yes." "Look," Nebuchadnezzar said, "I see four men loose and walking in the midst of the fire, and they are not hurt and the form of the fourth man is like the Son of God." Can you imagine the praise that went up by these three men! The Bible says that the fire had no power over their bodies and the hair on their heads was not singed, nor were their garments affected, and the smell of fire was not on them. What a wonderful God we serve. He can deliver on time (Daniel 3:19-27).

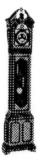

9. **Faithful to the End** - Of course, we all know that breast cancer claims many women's lives every year. But we must remember that we are on loan to each other in this world. This world is not our home. When God calls us home, it can be for many reasons. Everyone has their "season" to leave this world. Live your life to the fullest. Trust God to guide your footsteps. But most of all, accept Jesus Christ as your personal Savior so that when the time comes to leave this world, you'll stand waiting to hear, "Well done, my good and faithful servant, well done!" Picture me faithful Jesus!

10. **Healing Through Thought** - Writing this book was very much a part of the healing process for me. With every thought and written word, I felt deliverance. I hope these words will uplift someone through a bad day and encourage another having a good day. Jesus is a healer and He loves every woman unconditionally. Take Him at His Word. Trust Him without a doubt!

God Bless You All. Remember me in prayer as I am praying for all my sisters living through this disease.

SAS

I Shall Not Die, But Live
And Declare the Works of the Lord!

I shall not die, but I shall live,
And declare the works of the Lord!
I shall not sway from my belief,
My God won't pass me by.
His love is present every day,
We were born to live.
This earthly body may pass away,
But my soul was born to live.
Trust God for this life on earth,
Believe in everlasting life.
Above the stars and past the moon,
We all must take a flight.
Lord, make my journey quick and safe,
Lead me straight to Jesus Christ!

Rain

Tear drops from Jesus, life to the Earth,
Raindrops from Heaven, how much are they worth?
Rain down from Heaven, into my life,
Rinse away my troubles, clean up my life.
When my life is over, what is it worth?
Eternal life in Heaven, rain down on Earth.
Rain down on me Jesus, I know what it's worth,
Life everlasting, away from the Earth.

Looking in the Mirror

About 2-1/2 years ago, I was very sick.
The doctor said I had the C word,
I went through with no regrets.
The fear of C awaited:
Losing weight, losing hair, losing faith,
Oh, but I serve a powerful Jesus,
His love for me showed daily.
And it's still showing today,
For when I look in the mirror,
I see the Lord's Grace.
Thank you Jesus, for blessing me,
Day by day.
Grace overflowing,
All over my face.
(Hallelujah!)
(Praise the Lord!)

In the Middle of the Night

God moves in me, in the middle of the night.
When everything is quiet, the time is right.
He's waiting to tell me, He's standing with me.
I feel His presence, all around me.
The Holy Spirit covers me, from head to toe.
Anointing my spirit, to and fro.
Anoint me Jesus, move in my spirit - touch my soul,
Show me my journey on the earth.
So when this life is over, and it's time to start anew,
I know you'll be waiting, in the middle of the night.

Black Women of Strength

Connie and Bev,
Betty and Stachia,
Cathy Mc. And Darlene,
Brenda G. and Paula,
Lydia and Tina,
Thelma and Ruth,
Hollie and Shirley,
Mildred and Mary Lou,
Barbara and Cynthia,
Leomer and Gwen
Strength from first to last.
When my burden seems heavy,
And my prayers have been said,
Jesus always shows me Black women of strength.
Up above I've mentioned,
The pillars of strength in my life.
Love overflowing, rivers of tears,
Thank you Jesus for my pillars,
Black women of strength.

Listening

Listening means hearing,
Hearing means sensing,
Sensing means loving,
Loving means Jesus.
Thank you Jesus,
For listening to my problems,
Hearing my prayers,
Sensing my needs,
Caring enough to love me,
Unconditionally.

Listen sweet Jesus, listen.

Waking

Exactly what is waking?
Is it the opening of my eyes?
Is it knowing I'm taking a breath?
Is it the wiggling of my toes?
Exactly what is waking?
Waking is being in God's presence.
Waking is knowing God has opened my eyes.
Waking is knowing God has allowed me to take a breath.
Waking is knowing God is controlling my body and soul -
wiggling my toes.
Praise God for waking each and every day!

Attitude

Attitude is the way you think about something.
Good thoughts, bad thoughts,
Soon it will show through.
If you retain anger,
It will soon creep out,
Constantly making you hold back a shout.
God wants us happy - no attitudes,
Just think what your life would be like,
If God constantly had an attitude with you.
No grace, no peace, no mercy in sight.
Thinking about this, brings up fright.
I would be afraid if I knew,
God had an attitude with me.
Trust Him for grace, peace, love and mercy,
Remember to pray.

Aunt Sheila, Are You Going to be All Right?

When I awoke from my biopsy, the first person I saw,
Was my very special loved one, my nephew DeShawn.
Concern in his eyes, and love in his heart,
The question was asked, straight from the heart.
"Will you be all right?" my nephew asked,
With worry in his eyes, my reply was fast.
Yes, Shawn, I'll be all right, trust God, I said,
Everything's all right, I believe we both were blessed.

When Shawn asked this question, I didn't know his time was
winding up. Thank you Jesus for memories.

Marvel at the Magnitude of God

God is so large, He covers all space.
In Heaven and Earth, He's all over the place.
When you need a touch, wherever you are,
You can call on Him, He's both near and far.
Marvel at His magnitude, give Him the praise,
Both near and far, He covers all space.
So if you're having a bad day, or your fears have escalated,
Breathe God into your spirit, reach to your right or left.
Expect a breath from Heaven, and a touch right here on Earth.

Healing

Healing comes in many ways, I didn't know until now,
How God can send a healing, showering down.
Sickness, pain, and sorrow, all need a special touch,
When God sends a healing, you feel a gentle touch.
Soft words from Jesus, at fearful times,
Take away my sorrows, remove my fears,
I heard a word from Jesus, in the shower one day.
It seems He likes to deal with me in water.
God said it's over today.

(I believe God has delivered me from breast cancer. God said
it, I believe it.)

A Time and a Season

As time goes on, I must admit,
Life moves so fast, the seasons seem a myth.
From winter to spring, to summer and fall,
My God has a special time, for each season to call.
When we need a harvest, He sends the rain.
When the germs are roaring, He sends the cold air.
To protect us from germs, in the air.
As February ends, spring begins to blossom,
Telling us that God, is ever so awesome.
By the end of May, the temperature is rising,
Sunshine and fun, time is on the run.
By September the kids are back in school,
Such an instant change, that's the Golden Rule.
Waiting for your season, it won't be long,
Blink your eye, take in a deep breath, wait for God to call.

It Wasn't the Fiery Furnace, But it was Something I had to go Through!!

The anointing was upon me,
I could feel His presence near,
That special love of Jesus,
His Spirit was lingering near.
He held my hand and pulled me through,
At that moment, I knew,
It wasn't the fiery furnace,
But it was something I had to go through!!
Maybe you've been in trouble,
Maybe you are going through,
Reach out and hold tight,
God's spirit is covering you.
Remember we don't know what's coming,
But He's there to see you through,
Don't stop in the middle,
You've got to make it through.
It may not be the fiery furnace,
But it's something you have to go through.

SAS
"97"

What Do You Have in Your House to Give

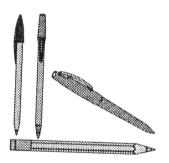

Sometimes we think God's looking for much,
When all He wants is your trust.
The widow woman came to Him,
Empty-handed, she thought she had nothing to give.
A debt she owed, no way to pay,
God said, "Give me what you have - invest and follow my instructions today!"
She gathered the empty vessels and filled them with oil,
God said, "Worry no more - close the door."
Sometimes I feel like the woman with the oil,
Instead of oil, it was pencil, paper, and pen.
The thoughts He's given me to express from within.
Have anointed my ink pen - again and again.
Ask me what I have in my house to give,
Thoughts of glory to God, again and again!
God said, "Worry no more - close the door!!"

II Kings 4:1-7

SAS
"97"

My Brother Adrian Gregory

My brother Adrian sometimes seems unreal to me,
We were born nine years apart.
He was much older than me.
By the time I was nine,
He was off to the service.
Coming home for holidays,
Leaving shortly, back to the service.
Sometimes it seems I really didn't have a brother.
He left us so early.
Lord, please have my brother,
I know he's worthy.
At 16 years old,
I knew little about salvation.
Adrian had to live fast and in a hurry,
Because Jesus was calling.
I remember my dad writing in his obituary:
"My son's come full circle,
Jesus, I pray you told him,
Come unto me and rest."

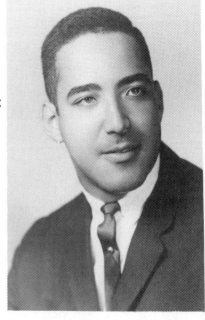

In Loving Memory of my Brother:
Adrian Anthony Gregory:
Oct 9, 1947 - March 26, 1972

When the Death Angel Stops By

The death angel came early in June,
He came to move Shawn early in June,
From one house to another, I couldn't understand why.
Because Jesus sent him on a journey, he had to stop by.
Early in the morning, a distressing call came.
Telling us the death angel had stopped to take DeShawn away.
From one house to another, I couldn't understand.
But Jesus knew his journey here, had come to an end.
Shawn flew with the angel, it didn't take long,
From one house to another, Shawn entered at God's throne.
We all must be ready, when the death angel stops by,
Get your house in order, get ready to fly.

Dedicated to my loving nephew.
DeShawn Jackson: March 7, 1975 - June 11, 1995

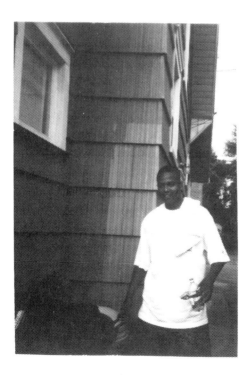

About

the

Author

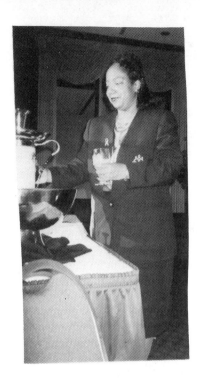

Sheila A. Gregory Stover was born in Canton, Ohio on
May 24, 1955. She is the daughter of Mr. and Mrs. Robert E.
Gregory. She graduated from McKinley High School in 1973
and Aultman School of Radiologic Technology in 1975.

Sheila married Anthony D. Stover on May 26, 1979. They
have three children: Tiana Renee, 15, Adrian Anthony, 11,
and Aaron Gregory 6.

Sheila is a member of the Antioch Baptist Church and
Rev. Richard L. Jordan is her pastor. She is a born again
Christian, breast cancer survivor, mammographer, and writer.

Sheila's favorite scriptures are:
- I shall not die, but live, and declare the works of the Lord!
- I can do all things through Christ, who strengthens me.
- Only what you do for Christ will last.

And her favorite saying is:
- Hold fast, the wind's blowing (see poem on back cover).

JOB

The God You Can Trust

Bryson Smith

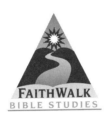

FAITHWALK
BIBLE STUDIES

CROSSWAY BOOKS • WHEATON, ILLINOIS
A DIVISION OF GOOD NEWS PUBLISHERS

15	14	13	12	11	10	09	08	07	06	05	04	03	02	01	00
15	14	13	12	11	10	9	8	7	6	5	4	3	2	1	

Contents

How to Make the Most of These Studies

1. What Is an Interactive Bible Study?

These "interactive" Bible studies are a bit like a guided tour of a famous city. The studies will take you through Job, pointing out things along the way, filling in background details, and suggesting avenues for further exploration. But there is also time for you to do some sightseeing on your own—to wander off, have a good look for yourself, and form your own conclusions.

In other words, we have designed these studies to fall halfway between a sermon and a set of unadorned Bible study questions. We want to provide stimulation and input and point you in the right direction, while leaving you to do a lot of the exploration and discovery yourself.

We hope that these studies will stimulate a lot of interaction—interaction with the Bible, with the teaching material, with your own ideas, with other people in discussion, and with God as you talk to Him about it all.

2. The Format

Each study focuses on a slice of Job and contains teaching material to introduce, summarize, suggest, and provoke. Interspersed throughout the teaching are three types of "interaction," each with its own symbol:

STARTING OUT

Questions to help you think about society and your own experience in a way that tunes you in to the issues being raised by the Bible passage.

FINDING TRUTH

Questions to help you investigate key parts of the Bible.

GOING FURTHER

Questions to help you think through the implications of your discoveries.

When you come to one of these symbols, you'll know that it's time to do some work on your own.

3. Suggestions for Individual Study

▲ Before you begin, pray that God will open your eyes to what He is saying in His Word and give you the strength to do something about it. You may be spurred to pray again at the end of the study.

▲ Work through the study, following the directions as you go. Write in the spaces provided.

▲ Resist the temptation to skip over the *Starting Out, Finding Truth,* and *Going Further* sections. It is important to think about the sections of text (rather than just accepting them as true) and to ponder the implications for your life. Writing these things down is a valuable way to get your thoughts working.

▲ Take what opportunities you can to talk with others about what you've learned.

4. Suggestions for Group Study

▲ Much of what we have suggested above applies to group study as well. The studies are suitable for structured Bible study or cell groups, as well as for more informal pairs and threesomes.

Get together with one or more friends and work on the studies at your own pace. You don't need the formal structure of a "group" to gain maximum benefit.

▲ It is vital that group members work through the study themselves *before* the group meets. The group discussion can take place comfortably in an hour (depending on how sidetracked you get!), but only if all the members have done the work and are familiar with the material.

▲ Spend most of the group time discussing the "interactive" sections—*Starting Out, Finding Truth,* and *Going Further.* Reading all the text together would take too long and should be unnecessary if group members have done their preparation. You may wish to underline and read aloud particular paragraphs or sections of text that you think are important.

▲ The role of the group leader is to direct the course of the discussion and try to draw the threads together at the end. This will mean a little extra preparation—underlining important sections of text to emphasize, deciding which questions are worth concentrating on, being sure of the main thrust of the study. Leaders will also probably want to decide approximately how long they'd like to spend on each part.

▲ We haven't included an "answer guide" to the questions in the studies. This is a deliberate move—we want to give you a guided tour of Job, not a lecture. There is more than enough in the text we have written and the questions we have asked to point you in what we think is the right direction. The rest is up to you.

▲ For more input, see "A Special Note for Discussion Leaders" at the end of the book.

1

Good Times, Bad Times

JOB 1–2

Workers dropped a crate containing a 75 million-year-old dinosaur skeleton outside a museum in The Hague, Netherlands, breaking it into 188 pieces. "The two Canadian scientists who had spent two years gluing together the skeleton had tears in their eyes," a spokesman told a *De Telegraph* reporter.
—*The Bulletin*, October 7, 1997

Most of us know what it's like to have one of *those* days. A day when nothing goes right and everything goes wrong. Sometimes those sorts of days are nothing more than a nuisance, and given time we can think back and laugh. Sometimes those days are far more tragic. The day the biopsy test comes back positive. The day the knock at the door is the police to tell you about a fatal accident. The day you discover a terrible secret within a relationship. Such days can be the start of unimaginable grieving and suffering.

The Old Testament book of Job takes us into the life of a man who loses virtually everything in a single day. Job's possessions, livelihood, children, and health are all ripped away in tragic circumstances. And Job is crippled by mind-numbing anguish.

On one level, therefore, the book of Job is all about suffering. It offers certain insights into why bad things happen. However, it is important to note from the outset that this is *not* the main focus of the book. As we'll discover, Job isn't really about *why* suffering happens. It's more about how we should act toward God *when* suffering happens.

In this respect Job is much more practical than theoretical. It's a bit like a first-aid manual. A first-aid manual doesn't really go into great detail about all the different reasons why you might break your arm. It is more geared toward explaining how to act when your arm is broken. That's like Job. It doesn't give us an exhaustive catalog of reasons *why* suffering happens; it is more concerned to explain how to act toward God *when* suffering happens.

Job is a book about whether God is worth following even when we are suffering. It's about whether God is worth trusting even when He seems to be making our life miserable.

But first things first. Let's meet the man Job and discover a bit about him.

 FINDING TRUTH

Read Job 1:1-5.

1. Describe Job's physical circumstances. He was very wealthy he had 7 sons a 3 daughters 7,000 sheep 3,000 camels 500 yoke of oxen 500 she donkeys and great numbers of work animals

2. Describe Job's character. His children often had parties and he would rise early and send for them to santify them and offer holocausts for each of them for they may have sinned against God

3. Read Proverbs 3:1-8. According to this passage, how are Job's wealth and blamelessness linked?

   By Keeping Gods commands and not relying on his own wisdom or pride but by always giving Glory to God he will not forget you Fear God and avoiding Evil

Job the Man

In these opening verses we are left in no doubt that Job is a godly man. We see this especially in the way that he is concerned not just for his own relationship with God but also for his family. He even offers sacrifices to God just in case his children have done something silly (1:5). This man is a model of loving concern. He is presented as the perfect example of a godly, wise man.

Job is also astronomically wealthy. He owns 7,000 sheep, 3,000 camels, 500 yoke of oxen, and 500 donkeys. Job is the Bill Gates of ancient Edom!

All of this is exactly what we would expect from what we read in Proverbs 3. As we've discovered in the above questions, Proverbs predicts that if you "fear the Lord and shun evil" you will be healthy, wealthy, and wise. Job feared the Lord and shunned evil, and he was healthy, wealthy, and wise. So far everything fits perfectly. Everything is as it should be. Everything is as we would want it: a good man enjoying a good life.

But that is all about to change. Some bad things are about to happen to this good man.

 FINDING TRUTH

Read Job 1:6-22.

1. What is Satan's accusation against Job?
   That A Man of his wealth and prosperaty. Why would he not praise the Lord and be dudtyful.

2. How does God respond? *He said to satan that all things are in satans power over Job but do not lay a hand on him and brings him bodily harm.*

3. What do we learn about God and Satan in these verses?
   That there is a kind of rivalry between them. That Satan wants God's Power. That he needs to find a way to take away the Love of God from his people.

4. What does God allow Satan to do to Job? What different types of events does Satan use to bring suffering to Job?

   Everything is taken away from Job. His Family is killed. All of his livestock are taken away His livelyhood is taken away. His workers but a few are killed.

5. How does Job respond?

He tears his cloths off in agany and throus his self down on the floor. And then praises God.

Job's First Test

In the space of a few minutes, Job loses everything. His wealth, his oxen, his sheep, his camels, his servants, his precious children whom he worried over so much; they are all gone—ripped away from him by both natural disasters and human violence.

The reason for Job's suffering is revealed to us, the readers, if not to Job. Satan has come before God and questioned Job's righteousness. Satan argues that Job follows God only for what Job can get out of it. According to Satan, Job is not really interested in God at all. Job just likes the gifts that God gives; and if the gifts were to suddenly disappear, says Satan, then Job would curse God.

In one sense this is a slur against Job's character, but it is also a slur against God. Satan is suggesting that God can only win friends for Himself by giving them things. He is suggesting that God has to buy followers with bribes and prizes.

The story progresses, with God accepting Satan's challenge, and it would seem by the end of chapter 1 that Satan has been proved wrong. After losing his prosperity and family, Job does not do what Satan predicted he would do. Just the opposite—rather than curse God, Job praises Him.

Satan, however, remains unconvinced.

 FINDING TRUTH

Read Job 2.

1. In this chapter, what further things do we discover about God, Satan, and Job?

   a. God *That he is sure that Job Loves him for himself. Not for the gifts that he gives or the wealth of family. That is why he gives Satan the power to harm but not Kill Job.*

b. Satan *That he is jealous of Job's Love for God. That he thinks that is Job suffers great physical pain that he will condem God and curse him.*

c. Job *That he is faithful to God he even tells his wife, Do we not accept the good that God gives us then we must also accept the evil things that they receive as well*

2. To what extent does Job understand why he is suffering?

That by being a servant of God that you take the Good & the Bad. If you praise God you do it always through whatever circumstances you are in that Does not change your relationship with God.

Job's Second Test

By the end of chapter 2, Job has gone from prosperity to poverty, from great comfort to crippling pain, from being the greatest man among all the people of the East to sitting on a rubbish pile scratching his scabs with a broken piece of pottery.

In all this, it is crucial to notice that Job has not been aware of the discussion between Satan and God. Job knows nothing about what has happened in heaven. He knows only that he is suffering. Indeed, much of the remainder of the book is taken up with Job arguing with his friends and struggling with God over why these terrible things have happened to him.

For us the readers, though, the issue is slightly different. Unlike Job, we do know why he is suffering. We are told in the first eleven verses! Job is suffering as a test of his righteousness. For us the readers, the real tension of the book is whether or not Job will remain faithful amid his suffering. Will Job's despair cause him to curse God? Will Satan be proved right?

In the studies that follow we will discover how Job handles his sufferings. As we do so, the question that will pop up time and time again is, How should *we* respond to God when bad things happen to us and we don't understand why?

 GOING FURTHER

1. When we suffer, do you think it is usually for the same reason that Job suffered?

   I don't normally Look at it that way but that is the reason that we all suffer. It is at the hand of Satan not God For God is our Father and Loves us.

2. Satan accuses Job of being more interested in God's gifts than in God Himself. To what extent could this be true for you? In what ways can we ensure that we don't fall into that trap?

   It would be easy to look at all that God has given me my family home job etc. and take that for granted. But I need to always remember that those are Gifts that God has given to me and to Praise Him in All things

3. In what ways is God's sovereignty revealed in these opening chapters?

   Where it says that one day the Sons of God came to present themselves to the Lord. That is showing God is King the Ruler. It doesn't say God Presented himself to the Angels does it.

4. When is it hard to believe that God is in control?

When we look at All the things happening day in and day out we may find it hard that Satan hasen't taken over. All you need do is to watch the news read the paper and watch a great portion of our Entertainment TV Movies Music magazines & books to see the Course that people have Choosen and that it is Contrary to Gods Ways

5. When we are suffering, how can it be comforting to remember that God is in control?

That God will never give you more than you Can handle, At the time it may be overwelhming, but that is because we are looking at the whole things and wondering how we can fix it! As time goes on we need to realize that we can't fix 1 little bit of it. That we ourselves are unable to do it alone. With God All things are possible. That as we anilize and look at the situation we break it down into different parts, we take it apart like a puzzle. that we work on and put together one piece at a time. It doesnt Mean that we can no longer feel the pain it just isn't always to the point where it is All Consuming We are able with Gods Grace to take it one step at a time. Work on it little by little

DONNA & FAMILY   BETH Denise

Randy Bob & Family Michael - beths brother

Mark - beths cousins Beths Mom & Dad

Joyce's Friend - Helen - care receiver - Danny

Lori & Baby Janiers Uncle Butch & Aunt Gisela

Nancy & Barb

Mom & Dad (Billcole's Family)

Birthday Party on Oct 5th
For (Donna & Beth)

Bring Cover Dish
at Donna's

2

Life Is Never That Simple

JOB 3–27

Nothing comes from nothing, nothing ever could.
Somewhere in my youth or childhood
I must have done something good.

Do you recognize those words from Rodgers and Hammerstein's *The Sound of Music*? Do you remember the scene? Maria is back after having run away, all the children are happy again, Captain von Trapp has called off his engagement to the Baroness, and Maria and the Captain have finally declared their love for each other. All is well with the world. Everyone in the audience is feeling warm and fuzzy. And Maria sings that, somewhere in her youth or childhood, she must have done something good to deserve this moment.

Is that the way life operates? Is that the secret to getting on in the world? That if we do good things, then good things will happen to us; and if we do bad things, bad things will happen to us? Is that how it works?

Many of us instinctively think so. When something goes wrong, often our immediate response is, "What have I done to deserve this? Am I being punished for something?" In some Christian circles this sort of thinking is reinforced with very spiritual-sounding reasons. People are told that the reason they are sick or in trouble is that they have some unconfessed sin in their life. They are told that if they confess their sin and repent, then things will get better.

But is that the way life works? That is the question we'll be investigating in this study.

FINDING TRUTH

1. Read Job 2:11-13. What do Job's three friends do in response to his suffering? What does this tell us about his friends?

2. Read Job 3. What does Job say to his friends about his own suffering? How does this compare with what Satan predicted in 2:5?

Job's Comforters

In our last study we left Job sitting in ashes, scratching the scabs that covered his body from head to foot. Three friends of Job now arrive, and they are so horrified by what they see that for a whole week they sit in silence. It is Job who breaks the silence, with a sad lament of his birth (chapter 3). This is all the invitation the friends need to now speak for themselves, and for the next thirty chapters a huge debate develops between Job and his friends, as they argue about why all this has happened to Job.

In one sense, the structure of Job simply mirrors life. In a chapter and a half, Job loses everything, but then for the next thirty chapters there is endless soul-searching, grieving, arguing, and wondering why. That is so much like life. A five-minute phone call can bring your whole life crashing down, but the grieving and confusion can go on for months if not years.

Unfortunately, it is at this stage of the book that many readers lose interest, for as the discussion between Job and his friends develops, it becomes somewhat repetitive and (to us) long-winded. Job's three friends each take turns at explaining to Job why he is suffering. After each friend has had his say, Job himself replies to him before the next friend speaks. This entire pattern then repeats itself two more times. All this can be represented by the following table:

Round 1	Chapters
Eliphaz speaks, Job responds	4–7
Bildad speaks, Job responds	8–10
Zophar speaks, Job responds	11–14
Round 2	
Eliphaz speaks, Job responds	15–17
Bildad speaks, Job responds	18–19
Zophar speaks, Job responds	20–21
Round 3	
Eliphaz speaks, Job responds	22–24
Bildad speaks, Job responds	25–26
. . . . Job responds	27–31

It can be seen that the discussion runs out of steam toward the end, with Zophar not even offering a third speech. We'll say more about this later. For the remainder of this study we will be dipping into some of the things that Job's first two friends say. In our next study, we'll look at Zophar, and then finally at what Job himself thinks.

So then, what words of comfort do Job's friends offer?

 FINDING TRUTH

1. Read Eliphaz's first speech (Job 4–5).

    a. How would you describe the tone of Eliphaz's speech? Is he supportive? Cruel? Caring? Understanding?

b. What does Eliphaz think is the reason behind Job's sufferings? (4:7-8)

c. Why is Eliphaz so confident about his assessment of Job? (4:12-16)

d. What is Eliphaz's advice to Job? (5:8, 17)

2. Look now at Eliphaz's last speech (chapter 22). Is he still saying the same things?

3. Read Job 8:1-7.
    a. What does Bildad think is the reason behind Job's suffering?

    b. What does Bildad think Job should do to restore his blessings?

4. Looking back over the advice of Eliphaz and Bildad:

    a.   What do they have in common?

    b.   In what ways are they different?

Nothing Comes from Nothing?

Despite some variations in emphasis, Eliphaz, Bildad (and Zophar) all agree that Job's suffering is the result of unconfessed sin. God is just, they argue; good people don't have bad things happen to them; therefore, Job must have done something wrong to deserve the trouble he is experiencing. You almost expect Job's three friends to break out into a variation of the song mentioned earlier: "Nothing comes from nothing. Nothing ever could. So somewhere in your youth or childhood, Job, you must have done something bad."

We will consider Job's responses to his friends in study 4; suffice it to say that Job denies their accusations. Job knows of no sin bad enough to warrant the degree of suffering he is going through. This leads to a great impasse in the debate. Job's friends cannot get Job to confess his sin, and Job cannot convince his friends that there is nothing to confess!

The frustration for us, the readers, is that we know that Job's friends are wrong. Ever since the very first verse of the book we have known that Job is a blameless and upright man who fears God and shuns evil. We've heard it from God's own lips when He was talking to Satan (1:8). What this alerts us to is that suffering can happen to anyone, even to those who don't deserve it. In this fallen world, sometimes even the innocent can suffer.

Job's friends have failed to appreciate this because their theology is too precise and their view of God too small. Job's friends make the mistake of reducing God to virtually an impersonal system of cause and effect. In their view of the world, good things happen to good people; bad things happen to bad people—simple as that. The result is that, although much of what they say about God is true, it isn't the complete truth about God. In the end their counsel, though well-meaning, is both naive and cruel.

Jesus and Undeserved Suffering

Job alerts us to the reality that undeserved suffering can happen in this life. Although none of us is perfect, bad things can still happen that are not the direct result of some sin we have committed. This of course raises the issue of why God allows such things to happen. And as we'll see, this is exactly the question on Job's lips.

However, we must not forget what we discovered in our first study: The book of Job is most interested not in *why* seemingly undeserved suffering happens, but in *how to respond* to God when it does happen.

In this respect Jesus Christ stands as our supreme example:

> *For it is commendable if a man bears up under the pain of unjust suffering because he is conscious of God. . . . To this you were called, because Christ suffered for you, leaving you an example that you should follow in his steps.*
>
> *"He committed no sin, and no deceit was found in his mouth."*
>
> *When they hurled their insults at him, he did not retaliate; when he suffered, he made no threats. Instead, he entrusted himself to him who judges justly.*
>
> —1 Peter 2:19, 21-23

GOING FURTHER

1. What can we learn from Job's friends concerning helping each other through suffering?

2. What do the following passages have to say about possible reasons for suffering?

   ▲ Luke 13:1-5

   ▲ John 9:1-3

   ▲ 1 Corinthians 11:27-32

   ▲ Hebrews 12:7-11

3. Imagine that a friend is going through a great personal tragedy, and someone tells him that his suffering is because of an unconfessed sin in his life. What might you say in response to that idea?

4. What do you think it means to "entrust" yourself to "him who judges justly" (1 Pet. 2:23)? What practical ways can we help each other do this?

3

Where's the Justice?

JOB 20–21

For the thirsty, there is nothing more agonizing than seeing someone else with a tall, cool glass of refreshment. For the lonely, there is nothing more heartbreaking than seeing someone else really enjoying a relationship. And for those who are suffering unjustly, there is nothing more galling than seeing the wicked prospering.

 STARTING OUT

1. Can you think of any current examples where you see the wicked or ungodly "getting away with it"?

2. How does it make you feel when you see that happening?

In our last study, we saw how Job's friends tried to "comfort" him by urging him to repent. "Your suffering must be due to some sin," they helpfully pointed out. "And since we know that God is just, all you need to do is turn back to Him and He'll restore you to your former glory."

The only problem is that Job has nothing to repent of. Job knows this, and we, the readers, know it too (because we were privy to the conversation between God and Satan in chapter 1). But Job's friends just can't accept it. Zophar, in particular, is adamant that God would not be so unjust as to punish anyone unless he or she is among the wicked.

Let's look at Zophar's second and final speech, and at Job's stinging reply.

 FINDING TRUTH

Read Job 20:1-7.

1.   According to Zophar:

    a.   What is the current state of the wicked?

    b.   What does the future hold for them?

2.   What is Zophar's basis for saying this?

3. Read Job 20:12-29.

    a.   What reason(s) does Zophar give for the eventual downfall of the wicked?

    b.   How do you think Job would hear this? What does it say to him?

4. Now read Job 21. How would you summarize Job's answer to Zophar?

5. Why is all this particularly hard for Job to take?

Why Do the Wicked Prosper?

Zophar continues the theme that all three of Job's friends have been pursuing since the beginning of their conversation; namely, that in God's world good people get good things and bad people get bad things—simple as that. His lengthy catalog of the miseries that will come upon the wicked is hardly what you could call sensitive counseling. It serves as a very blunt accusation. Since Job is experiencing exactly the sort of horrors that always come upon the wicked, what does that make Job?

Job's answer is simply to point out the obvious: Anyone with any experience of the world knows that there are plenty of wicked people who don't seem to be suffering the terrible punishments Zophar has listed. "Just look around," says Job. "Can't you see many wicked people living in comfort and ease, with their children around them? Where's the justice in that?"

This is an important question, one that we often grapple with and that the Bible often addresses. Why is it that evil and corrupt people seem to prosper, and the righteous very often do not?

Let us investigate further to see what light we can shed on this age-old question.

 FINDING TRUTH

1. Read Job 24:21-25.

    a. In what sense does Job agree with Zophar about the wicked?

    b. Where, then, does he disagree with Zophar?

2. Read Psalm 37:1-11.

    a. How is this similar to what Zophar is saying?

    b. How is it different?

3.   Read Hebrews 11:32-40.

    a.   What did the heroes of the Old Testament have in common?

    b.   How did they respond to hardship and suffering?

Getting It Right

When we compare Zophar's argument with the rest of the Bible, and indeed with what Job also says, we can see that Zophar is half right. The wicked will certainly get what they deserve—eventually. But that "eventually" may take some time, and in the meantime the righteous must wait patiently, believing and trusting in God.

This is where Zophar's logic comes unstuck. The wicked will one day be judged by God and will suffer. But the fact that certain people suffer does not automatically mean they are wicked; and the fact that certain people prosper does not automatically mean they are righteous. That Job is suffering is not an indication that he is automatically to be numbered among the wicked. He may well be a righteous man who needs to wait patiently for God to vindicate Him.

In fact, this is precisely the case with Job, whom God is allowing to suffer, not because of any wickedness on Job's part, but for His own secret purposes.

The right response to suffering and hardship is to patiently wait for God, to trust Him completely, to put our faith in Him. This is not easy to do, as Job is discovering. And seeing your ungodly neighbor living in ease and luxury doesn't make it any easier.

 GOING FURTHER

1.   From what you have read of Job so far, how would you rate Job's attitude toward his suffering?

2. When you see an ungodly or corrupt person prospering:

▲ How do you tend to react?

▲ How do you treat that person?

▲ What changes do you need to make in this area?

4

Why Me, God?

JOB 3–27

Late at night on August 31, 1997, Diana, Princess of Wales, was killed in a car accident in Paris. There followed an extraordinary outpouring of emotion around the world. Her funeral was the most-watched television event in history, with an estimated worldwide audience of 2.5 billion. Buckingham Palace and Kensington Palace were awash in an estimated $54 million worth of flowers.

As I sat at home watching all of this on television, one particular image stuck in my mind. It was a close-up shot of one of the bouquets outside Kensington Palace. Pinned to the flowers was a card with just one word on it: "Why?" That one word seemed to capture so many people's sentiments. Why do things like fatal car accidents happen? Why do beloved people die early in life? Why are young children left without a mother? Why are so many people around the world put through such grief?

Maybe there have been times of suffering in your life when you have asked the same question. "Why?" It is the question that Job asks God throughout chapters 3–27.

In study 2 we noted that Job 3–27 contains a long and rather repetitive discussion between Job and his three friends, Eliphaz, Bildad, and Zophar. Job's friends are convinced that Job's suffering must be the result of some unconfessed sin in Job's life. In this study, we will examine Job's responses to his friends' accusations.

 FINDING TRUTH

Read Job's first response to Eliphaz, in chapters 6–7.

1. How does Job describe his anguish? (6:1-7)

2. What does Job wish would happen to him, and why? (6:8-13)

3. How does Job feel about Eliphaz's advice? (6:14-30)

4. How does Job feel toward God? (7:11-21)

Job's Answer

In response to his friends' accusations, Job insists that he has not done anything to warrant his suffering. Job denies that there is some secret sin lurking in his life that has caused his distress. Job is not claiming to be perfect, simply that he has not done anything bad enough to warrant the degree of suffering he is going through.

This actually puts Job in a very frustrating situation. If Job's friends were correct, then his suffering could be more easily managed. It would be simply a matter of confessing and repenting of the sin, and then his good fortune would be restored. This is exactly what Eliphaz predicts could happen (5:17-27). But it's not that simple for Job. Job knows there is nothing to confess! All that is left for Job to do is to mourn the extent of his suffering (6:2-3), beg that God might shorten his life (6:8-9), and struggle over why God would bring such suffering upon him (7:20-21).

FINDING TRUTH

1. Read Job 9:1-20. What does Job seem to be saying of God here? What is Job's frustration?

2. Read Job 13:20-27. What does Job ask of God?

3. Read Job 19:23-29. How does Job express his confidence in God's justice?

4. Read Job 27:1-6.
    a. What does Job accuse God of doing?

    b. What is Job's attitude toward God in these verses?

c. How do Job's responses to his suffering compare with what Satan predicted in 1:11 and 2:5?

5. In study 2 we discovered that Job's friends had too small a view of God. They treated Him as an impersonal cause and effect. Are there any signs of this same attitude in Job?

Job's Frustration

In his suffering Job, like us, moves through a wide range of emotions. At times Job is so confident of God's justice that, even if a resurrection from the dead were required to vindicate him, then he believes it would happen (19:25-26)! At other times Job's despair causes him to question whether God would even give him a fair trial (9:14-17). As his bitterness grows, Job's language even drifts into disrespect toward God (27:2-6). We will return to consider this in a later study.

What is very noticeable, however, is Job's frustration at several levels. For starters, Job is in desperate need of a true friend. In 6:14 Job says that, "A despairing man should have the devotion of his friends, even though he forsakes the fear of the Almighty. But my brothers are as undependable as intermittent streams." Job's suffering is heightened by his loneliness. He desperately needs a friend who will stick by him, rather than the undependable friends he presently has. Better still, Job needs a friend who can empathize with him, someone who knows what it's like to be in his shoes, to suffer great loss for no apparent reason.

As well as a friend, Job would like to find an advocate to represent him before God. Job is well aware that God "is not a man like me that I might answer him, that we might confront each other in court." Therefore he needs "someone to arbitrate between us, to lay his hand upon us both" (9:32-33). Job is frustrated that God is so different from us. How on earth can we relate to the God of the universe? Job sees that he needs an arbitrator and mediator to bridge the gap between humanity and God.

Job needs a friend and a mediator. It's not too hard to see that Job needs Jesus.

 GOING FURTHER

1. Think back to a time when you have suffered. How did you feel toward God? In what ways were you similar to or different from Job?

2. Read Hebrews 4:14-16. Why is Jesus the perfect friend and arbitrator?

3. How would knowing Jesus have helped Job?

4. How does knowing Jesus help us when we suffer?

5

A Word about Wisdom

JOB 28

There are few things in the world more irritating than a traffic jam. There you are, sitting in your car going nowhere, achieving nothing.

That's the sort of feeling we have by the time we reach Job 28. The discussion between Job and his friends is going nowhere and seems to be achieving nothing. Job's friends are convinced that his suffering is the result of a secret, unconfessed sin, whereas Job maintains that no such sin exists. Neither side is budging. The discussion has reached a stalemate, so much so that Zophar can't even be bothered contributing to the debate anymore (see the diagram in study 2). No one is going anywhere.

It's at this point that chapter 28 blows through the book like a breath of fresh air. The chapter comes right in the center of Job's last speech to his friends. But the chapter doesn't sound as though it is Job who is speaking. The language seems almost too calm and objective for Job. And it doesn't sound like any of Job's friends for the same reasons. It is as if chapter 28 is a bit of a break from all the monotonous arguing. It bursts into the book with a fresh perspective that will help us understand the main lesson of the book.

Before we look at Job 28, however, let us recall some connections between Job and wisdom.

FINDING TRUTH

1. Read Proverbs 3:1-20. What does this chapter say about:

   a. the value of wisdom?

   b. the characteristics of a wise person?

   c. the results of a wise life?

2. Look back at Job 1:1-3. In what ways was Job portrayed as the perfect example of a wise man?

The Nature of Wisdom

It can be seen from Proverbs that when the Bible speaks of "wisdom," it is referring to something more than academic knowledge. Being wise is not simply being intellectually smart or getting good grades in school. Wisdom is practical knowledge. It is knowing how to get the most out of life. This is because wisdom taps into the principles and patterns of creation (Prov. 3:19-20). Wisdom is based on understanding how the world operates (because it is God's world) and therefore how best to live within it.

Let us discover now what Job 28 says about wisdom.

▲ FINDING TRUTH

1. Read Job 28:1-11.

    a. What things of value are these verses about?

    b. Where can they be found?

    c. In what ways are the achievements of human beings impressive?

2. Read Job 28:12-28.

    a. What thing of value is now being discussed? How does it compare with the precious things discussed in the earlier verses?

    b. Where can it be found? (v. 28)

    c. What does it mean to "fear" the Lord?

The Big Idea of Job

The climactic teaching of Job 28 is that wisdom comes from God. This makes sense. Since it is God who created everything, He more than anyone should know what is wise and what is foolish. Only God can truly know the best way to live within His creation. True wisdom is therefore to fear the Lord (v. 28). In other words, the best way to negotiate this life is by living in reverent submission to the One who made us.

Within Job, the importance of true wisdom takes on added dimensions. Coming as it does at the close of a debate about why Job is suffering, Job 28 emphasizes the idea that true wisdom is not a matter of knowing *why* suffering happens; rather, true wisdom is a matter of *knowing the God who knows why* suffering happens. The appropriate way to approach suffering is therefore not to seek an explanation for it but to seek to know God better through the experience.

Not only is this the climax of Job 28, it is also *the* lesson of the entire book of Job. The book revolves around the idea that, if we want to live this life to the full, it is not a matter of knowing why things happen; instead it is a matter of knowing the God who knows why things happen. The wise person cannot necessarily explain why everything in life happens, but the wise person is in a right relationship with God. This is a critically important lesson, which we will return to again and again in later studies. It is also a lesson that helps us understand how the book of Job points us forward to Jesus Christ.

 FINDING TRUTH

1. According to 1 Corinthians 1:18-25, what is God's wisdom? How is this different from what Jews and Greeks expect or desire?

2. According to Colossians 2:2-3, where is wisdom and knowledge found?

3. Compare Proverbs 3:19-20 with Colossians 1:15-20. What parallels are there between Jesus Christ and wisdom?

Jesus and Wisdom

So far Job has taken us into a fallen world where even the innocent suffer. It has raised the whole question of how we should behave toward God in such a world. Now in chapter 28 we learn that in this world of suffering the most important thing is not to know why we are suffering but to know and fear God, who is the source of all wisdom. This serves to highlight the importance of Jesus Christ, for it is through Jesus that we can most fully know God.

We have already seen that Jesus is the great biblical example of undeserved suffering (cf. 1 Pet. 2:19-23). However, in Jesus, and especially in His crucifixion, we also see the supreme example of God's wisdom, for in defiance of all worldly wisdom God chose to save people and bring them to know Him through the suffering and death of His Son on the Cross (1 Cor. 1:18–2:10). Through Jesus we are reconciled to God and enter into the fullness of life as God intended it (Col. 2:9-10). In Christ we can experience every spiritual blessing (Eph. 1:3), and we are able to enter into God's eternal kingdom, which will never fade or perish (1 Pet. 1:3-4). In Christ we also have everything we need to know for life and godliness (2 Pet. 1:3). These are wonderful truths. When we know Jesus, we are at the heart of God's plan and goal for His creation. This is why Jesus Christ is the wisdom of God.

 GOING FURTHER

1. Job 28 has introduced us to the idea that in this world of suffering the most important thing is not to know why we are suffering, but to seek to know God better while we are suffering. What are some ways in which suffering can help us know God better?

2. In 1 Corinthians 1 Paul refers to Jesus as "foolishness" to the Greeks and a "stumbling block" to the Jews. What does he mean by that? In what ways is Jesus still foolishness and a stumbling block to people today?

3. If Jesus is the wisdom of God, and knowing Jesus is so wonderful, why is it that we often feel the need for more than Him in our lives?

4. What are some practical ways that we can help each other remember the greatness of following Jesus?

5. "Blessed are you when people insult you, persecute you and falsely say all kinds of evil against you because of me" (Matt. 5:11). Why do Jesus' words make sense, given what we have discovered in this chapter about wisdom, suffering, and knowing God?

6

The Summing Up

JOB 29–37

In the lengthy courtroom drama that is the book of Job, we have reached the summing up. The two sides (Job and his friends) have traded speeches for many chapters, and now it is time to present the closing arguments.

Job sums up his feelings in chapters 29–31.

 FINDING TRUTH

1. Read Job 30:15–31:37. How would you summarize Job's feelings about:

   a. his suffering?

   b. himself and his actions?

   c. God?

2. Thinking back over Job's arguments and complaints:

    a.   What does he know for certain to be true?

    b.   What is he ignorant of?

A New Twist

Job is an unusual book, at least for modern readers. Its structure and style are not what we are used to at all. When 31:40 proclaims that "the words of Job are ended," we assume that the arguments and debates are finally over, and that now Job might receive an answer.

Yet in chapter 32 we get another surprising twist in this surprising book. A young man named Elihu steps forward. We don't know who he is or where he has come from, but it seems that he has been listening to the debate with growing frustration. He proceeds to deliver one of the longest speeches in the book, claiming to enlighten everyone with a superior argument.

Will Elihu at last have the answer to Job's problem?

 FINDING TRUTH

1.   Read Job 33:12-18. Job wants God to answer him; according to Elihu, how is God already speaking to Job?

2.   Read Job 34:1-15, 31-37. What is Elihu's opinion of Job and his situation?

3. Read Job 35:1-8; 36:1-9 and 37:14-24.

    a. How does Elihu describe God?

    b. How do these descriptions bear on Job's situation?

Still Waiting for an Answer

With all the confidence of a young man, Elihu claims to have the answer, for Job and for his three friends. To his credit, Elihu does bring in some new elements to the discussion (such as the idea that God communicates to us by dreams and visions and by sending calamity upon us), and he does speak at length about the majesty and might of God, who is far above our questioning.

Yet we are left at the end still waiting for the final resolution. For all his eloquence, Elihu still does not know what we, the readers, know about the events of chapter 1 and the real reason for Job's suffering.

And this is what life is like for us as well. Even though we know so much about so many things—even about God as He reveals Himself to us—yet much is hidden from us. We do not have access to all of God's plans and purposes. He is the potter; we are but the clay. "O the depth of the riches and wisdom and knowledge of God!" says Paul. "How unsearchable his judgments and how inscrutable his ways!" (Rom. 11:33, RSV).

We finish Job 37 still wondering how God Himself will resolve the tension. After all this debating, who is in the right? Will God justify Job or rebuke him? Will He restore Job's fortunes or punish him for his impudence?

For this, we must read on.

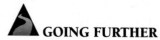 **GOING FURTHER**

1. List some things you know about:
   ▲ God

   ▲ the world

   ▲ your life

2. Now list some things that you *don't* know or understand about:
   ▲ God

   ▲ the world

   ▲ your life

3. What do you think your attitude should be toward:
   ▲ the things you do know and understand?

   ▲ the things you don't know or understand?

7

"Brace Yourself . . ."

JOB 38–41

The courtroom is full of people with anxious looks on their faces. The prosecution and the defense have summed up their cases, and the judge is about to hand down the decision. The hours of argument are now over. All that's left is to hear the verdict. But what will the verdict be? What will the judge decide? There is tension in the air.

That is the scene that greets us in Job 38–41. Much of the book to this point has been taken up in a painstaking argument between Job and his three friends, with the young Elihu as a late inclusion. Job has lost everything but his life, and his friends think that it is because of some unconfessed sin. Job, however, knows that this is not the case. So for chapter after chapter they have argued with each other, with no clear winner emerging.

But now it's time for the judge's verdict to be handed down. Brace yourself!

 FINDING TRUTH

To capture the majesty of God's speech, it is worthwhile to read what He says in full. Read Job 38–41.

1. Looking back over God's first speech (38:1–40:5):

   a. What is God's relationship to His creation?

b. What picture of God emerges?

c. Why do you think God speaks in this way?

d. What is the overall effect of the speech on Job?

2. At the conclusion of His first speech, God demands an answer from "the one who accuses God," that is, from Job (40:1-2). Job doesn't know what to say and offers no real answer at all. In response, God then begins a second speech, promising that "I will question you, and you shall answer me" (40:7).

   a. What is God's basic criticism of Job in 40:8-14?

   b. How does the material about the behemoth and the leviathan relate to this basic criticism? (See especially 41:10-11.)

3. Read Job's response to God's speech (42:1-5).

   a. What effect do God's speeches have on Job?

b. What exactly do you think Job is repenting of?

c. What good thing comes out of the way God speaks to Job?

God's Verdict

After thirty-eight chapters of debate about why Job is suffering, God finally speaks. And the surprising thing is what God *doesn't* say. God gives no reason whatsoever to Job as to why he is suffering. God does not tell Job anything about His conversation with Satan in chapters 1–2. Indeed, instead of giving answers to Job, God mainly asks questions, a crushing list of questions one after the other, all about nature. "Tell me, Job, can you shape the earth?" "Do you know where darkness lives?" "Can you move the stars around in the sky?" "Can you bring the rain to turn a desert into a grassland?" Can you do this? Can you do that? Question after question after question.

God's words have the effect of completely humbling Job. The questions remind Job of who is God and who isn't. Job is brought to repentance (42:6).

It is important to realize that Job is not repenting from any sins that caused his suffering; we have known from the opening chapter that Job's suffering is not a punishment for sin. It is not that his friends have been right all along and that there has been an unconfessed sin in his life. What, then, is Job repenting of?

During His long series of questions, God says of the leviathan, "No one is fierce enough to rouse him. Who then is able to stand against me? Who has a claim against me that I must pay? Everything under heaven belongs to me" (41:10-11). In the face of such reminders of God's greatness, Job realizes that he has been presumptuous and demanding toward God. He repents of the sin of not handling his suffering in the right way. He repents of "obscuring God's counsel" (cf. 42:3) and of demanding an explanation from God as if God owed him one.

All this teaches us two very valuable lessons. *First*, we are alerted to the danger of being too demanding with God. In Christ we enjoy great intimacy, boldness, and confidence with God, but we must be careful not to fall into the trap of taking God casually or flippantly. We must never forget that we are the creatures and He is the Creator. We have no right to question His ways or complain of His judgments. We belong to Him, like all of creation; we have no claim against Him that He must pay.

Even when we suffer—especially when we suffer—we must remember that perspective. Suffering can be a very crippling experience, and in the middle of pain and grief and loss our world can close in around us. We can become completely engrossed in our own selves and our problems. We can become quite selfish. But no matter how difficult things may be, it is never an excuse for being disrespectful or presumptuous with God. Certainly we may pour out our troubles to God. We can express to Him our confusion and sorrow about why He is doing something. But in our struggles with the hard questions of life we must never neglect the reverence and awe that God deserves. We need to remember our place. He is the Judge, not us. Job experienced more suffering than most of us could begin to imagine. He lost his family, his livelihood, and his health; and yet all that was still no excuse for inferring that God was unjust in allowing his suffering. It was no excuse for an attitude that demanded an answer from God, as if he were owed one.

But *second*, God's questions to Job show us that God's priority is to restore His relationship with Job rather than to explain to Job why he is suffering. God is more concerned that Job relate to Him properly, and submit to Him in all things, than that Job should know the answer to all things. This relates to the important lesson we discovered in study 5: "The fear of the Lord—that is wisdom" (Job 28:28). The key to wisdom, to making the best of life, is not to know why things happen; the key is to know the God who knows why things happen. That is what God seeks to do with Job. God's speeches have the effect of revealing God to Job. He now sees what God is like and fears God in a way that he never has before.

▲ GOING FURTHER

1. Read the following Bible passages and describe how they provide positive examples of how to relate to God during difficult times:

    ▲ Psalm 57

    ▲ Lamentations 3:19-33

    ▲ Habakkuk 3:17-19

    ▲ Luke 22:39-46

2. What practical things can we do to avoid becoming bitter when we suffer?

3. How does the picture God presents of Himself in chapters 38–41 compare with how He is often spoken of today:

   a. among non-Christians?

   b. among Christians?

4. In 42:2 Job says to God, "No plan of yours can be thwarted." How does this help us deal with suffering and relate rightly to God?

8

Faith, Mystery, and the Meaning of Life

JOB 42

In the United States it is now possible to watch "interactive" movies. Instead of simply sitting down and passively watching the movie, you are given a remote control device with which you can vote at various points throughout the movie on what you would like to happen next. So at certain critical points in the story line you use your remote control to cast a vote as to whether the bad guy gets caught yet, or whether you want the couple to say that they love each other, or whether you want the butler or the maid to be the murderer. Depending on what the majority of people in the audience vote for, the movie goes off in that direction. Only in America!

The voting patterns among audiences at these movies has led to an interesting discovery about human nature: People like happy endings! That's what audience after audience chooses—happy endings. We like it when people live happily ever after.

For this reason, the ending of the book of Job should please us.

 FINDING TRUTH

Read Job 42.

1. What is Job's response to God's speeches?

2. What does Job repent of?

3. What is God's opinion of Job's friends?

4. What exactly did Job's friends get wrong about God?

5. What happens to Job after he prays for his friends? How does his final state compare with how he started the book?

6. How do you feel at the end of the book? Happy? Confused? Surprised?

7. Are there any other things or people in the book of Job that you would like to know more about but that the ending doesn't tell you about?

And They All Lived Happily Ever After

Job has taken us into the world of a man who experiences unimaginable suffering. At the beginning of the book, and unknown to the human characters in the story, Satan claims that Job is a selfish man who only follows God for what he can get out of it. So to test Job, God gives Satan permission to make Job's life miserable, a task that Satan performs particularly well—Job loses everything.

It only adds to Job's suffering that he hasn't a clue as to why any of it has happened to him. Job's friends think they know why. They say that it's punishment for an unconfessed sin. But both we the readers and Job know that this is not the case. Finally, after what seems to be an endless debate between Job and his friends, God Himself appears. God doesn't tell Job why he has suffered or offer any explanation at all. Rather, God reminds Job of who is God and who isn't. God rebukes Job for demanding an answer as if God owed him one.

For virtually the entire book, most of us wouldn't swap places with Job for anything. His life is a mess, his children are gone, his health is in tatters, his wife is telling him to curse God and die, his friends are telling him to repent of a sin that he knows he hasn't committed, and God Himself is hauling Job over the coals for being disrespectful. And at the end of it all Job still doesn't know why his life has become so miserable.

Yet here at the end, halfway through the very last chapter, things suddenly turn good just as quickly as they had turned bad. Job has another family—seven more sons, three more daughters. No women are more beautiful than his daughters. Job becomes wealthier than he ever was. He gains herds twice the size of what he had before. Job himself lives to a ripe old age, seeing his children and their children to the fourth generation. Eventually Job dies, "old and full of years," which is a biblical epitaph reserved for the great ones such as Abraham and David.

So Job goes out with a very happy ending; except, as well as being a happy ending, it is also a little confusing. No reason is given for Job's return to good fortune. Is it a reward because he passed Satan's test? And what about Satan, anyway? God tells Job's friends that they have been in the wrong. But what about Satan? He was the one who started all the trouble in the first place! What does God say to him?

And what about Elihu? Elihu was the young fellow who had

kept quiet until chapter 32. He doesn't even rate a mention here at the end. God speaks to Job and to Job's three friends, but not a word to Elihu and not even a word *about* Elihu. The book ends without our even being sure who he was.

Job's ending may be happy, but it's also a little frustrating because of all the loose ends still dangling. We wish we were told more— which is exactly the point, because that's what life is like.

 GOING FURTHER

1. Think back over all the characters in the book. Every character to some extent didn't know or understand something.

   a. What did Satan not understand?

   b. What did Job not understand, even at the end of the book?

   c. What did Job's friends not understand, even at the end of the book?

   d. What did Elihu not understand?

   e. What do we the readers not know, even at the end of the book?

2. Who in the book is the one person who does know and understand everything?

3. What do you think the book of Job is telling us about life?

Life Is a Mystery

The book of Job is exactly like life. Both the book and life can be confusing and surprising at times. Unexpected bad things can happen. Unexpected good things can happen. Long periods of struggle and anguish and grieving can happen. And there are times in this life when we wish God would tell us more about what is going on.

Job wished God would tell him why he was suffering, but God never did. We wish God would tell us more about Elihu and what happened to Satan at the end, but God doesn't. It's frustrating that He doesn't, but that's just the way life is.

All this mystery serves only to reinforce the main lesson of Job. It is the lesson we learned in study 5—that if we want to live this life to the full, it's not a matter of knowing why things happen; it's a matter of knowing the God who knows why things happen.

The book of Job, like life, is full of confusing and surprising and sad and happy times, none of which we may ever fully understand. And the way through it all is not to try to figure out the meaning of every event. That's what Job's friends tried to do. They wanted to nail everything down and have all the answers. In the end, God condemned their attitude.

No, the wise way to live is not by knowing why everything happens, because we'll never achieve that. The way through the struggles and changes of life is to know the God who knows everything. The way to negotiate life is to know Jesus Christ.

For this reason, when bad or good things happen to us, the main question to grapple with is not, "Why is this happening to me?" The main question to consider is, "Since this is happening to me, how can I use it to know God better through Jesus Christ?"

This is what the book of Job has been about from start to finish. It is about staying close to God and trusting Him, even when bad things happen, because staying close to God is more valuable than the avoidance of suffering.

 GOING FURTHER

1. Why do we not value knowing God? What things do we tend to value more than knowing Him?

2. How might we know Jesus better when:

    a. a personal moral failure occurs?

    b. a tragedy causes great suffering?

c.   we become financially prosperous?

d.   we are in financial trouble?

e.   a close friend fails us?

3.   Look back over the studies in this book. Is there any one truth that has stood out to you? Why? What changes are you going to make in your life as a result of this truth?

A Special Note
For Discussion Leaders

Job presents its own particular problems for group Bible study, not the least of which is its length. Especially in the main body of the book (chapters 3–37), the long passages of discussion and debate are somewhat daunting. Reading these chapters in the group may be hard going, and so it is important to encourage each group member to read these sections beforehand. Even if the members are not doing any other preparation, try to get them at least to read the passages. It will help greatly in picking out what essentially is being said.

In terms of the content of the studies, it is likely that some discussion in the group will focus on God's sovereignty and how it relates to human responsibility and agency. Some may find it hard to come to terms with the absolute might and rule of God represented in Job, but in a sense that is the very point of the final five chapters of Job. You may need to allow extra time to discuss these questions (perhaps after study 7); you may find questions about election and predestination emerging as well. It may be worth taking an extra week and doing a topical study on these matters. *The Blueprint* contains a good introductory study on the topic.*

The other main issue to be aware of as a group leader is that group members may have differing experiences of suffering—either past or present. For some in the group, the puzzle of Job's sufferings and how to think about it may be largely an intellectual challenge; for others it may represent a very real and personal anguish, given their own suffering. You need to be sensitive to this possibility and respond appropriately (possibly outside of the group time).

The Blueprint is one of the Topical Bible Studies published by Matthias Media. It contains ten studies on different aspects of Christian doctrine, including the study "Who Is In Control?" which deals with God's sovereignty in creation, revelation, and redemption. To order, contact Matthias Media through their website: www.matthiasmedia.com.au.

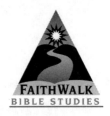

FAITHWALK
BIBLE STUDIES

Ask your local bookstore about these other
FaithWalk Bible Studies

Notes

About Matthias Media

This Bible study guide, part of the *FaithWalk Bible Studies,* was originally developed and published in Australia by Matthias Media. Matthias Media is an evangelical publisher focusing on producing resources for Christian ministry. For further information about Matthias Media products, visit their website at: www.matthiasmedia.com.au; or contact them by E-mail at: sales@matthiasmedia.com.au; or by fax at: 61-2-9662-4289.